613.25    Hutton, Lauren.
H
          The Slim-Fast body-
          mind-life makeover.

$24.00

| DATE | | | |
|---|---|---|---|
| | | | |
| | | | |
| | | | |
| | | | |
| | | | |
| | | | |
| | | | |
| | | | |
| | | | |
| | | | |
| | | | |
| | | | |
| | | | |

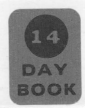

# THE Slim·Fast®

## BODY·MIND·LIFE
## MAKEOVER

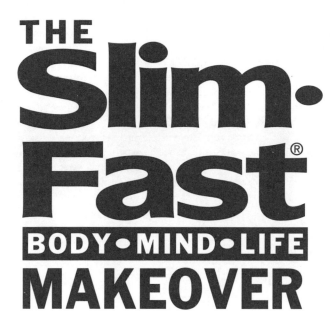

# THE Slim·Fast® BODY·MIND·LIFE MAKEOVER

# LAUREN HUTTON

## with Deborah Kotz

Foreword by David Heber, M.D., Ph.D.
Preface by George Blackburn, M.D., Ph.D.

ReganBooks
*An Imprint of HarperCollinsPublishers*

This book contains information relating to losing weight and weight maintenance. It is not intended to replace medical advice. Rather, the information provided should be used to supplement regular care by medical professionals.

Several particular warnings are in order: If you want to lose weight and are under eighteen, pregnant, nursing, following a diet recommended by a doctor, have health problems, or want to lose more than 30 pounds, see a doctor before starting the Slim•Fast program or any other weight-loss program. No one should lose more than 2 pounds a week after the first week on a weight-loss program. Rapid weight loss may cause health problems. The Slim•Fast products should *not* be used as a sole source of nutrition. You should eat at least 1,200 calories a day.

The testimonials included in this book may make reference to weight-loss results. These results are not typical and you should not necessarily expect to experience these results. Weight loss averages 1 to 2 pounds a week during the weight-loss period, after the initial week.

The author, the publisher, and the Slim•Fast Foods Company expressly disclaim responsibility for any adverse effects arising from following the diet or exercise program in this book without appropriate medical supervision.

Published under license from the Slim•Fast Foods Company.

Visit us at www.slim-fast.com.

HarperCollins books may be purchased for educational, business, or sales promotional use. For information please write: Special Markets Department, HarperCollins Publishers Inc., 10 East 53rd Street, New York, NY 10022.

FIRST EDITION

*Designed by Stanley S. Drate / Folio Graphics Co. Inc.*
*Illustrations on pages 257 to 275 by Durell Godfrey*
*Food photography by Tom Eckerle Studio*
*Styling by Roscoe Betsil and Ceci Gallini*
*Props courtesy of The Terence Conran Shop, NYC*
*Recipes by Suzanne Kokkins, Registered Dietitian*
*Diving photographs of Lauren © 2000 by Tanya Burnett*

Printed on acid-free paper.

Library of Congress Cataloging-in-Publication Data has been applied for.

ISBN 0-06-039335-1

00 01 02 03 04 ❖/RRD 10 9 8 7 6 5 4 3 2 1

# Contents

# Acknowledgments

Many people helped turn the Slim•Fast Makeover into this book. Special thanks go to the team of professionals from ReganBooks and HarperCollins: Charles Woods, Cassie Jones, and Carl Raymond are only a few of the talented individuals who made this book possible. Without Cal Morgan, the book's editor, this project would never have been completed. And, of course, a special thanks to Judith Regan, who believed in the potential of this book from the very beginning. Lauren's assistant, Carol Wood, has been crucial to the logistics of this complicated project.

And the many people of the Slim•Fast Foods Company deserve special recognition for their role in bringing this book to fruition—chief among them Dr. Harry Greene, who provided guidance every step of the way, and Jordan Herzberg, whose energetic supervision was critical to the book's success. Finally, the real credit for this book should go to the founder of Slim•Fast, Dan Abraham. For fifty years, Danny has been committed to reducing the ever-growing epidemic of obesity in the United States and encouraging a healthy, dynamic society. This book is as much as anything a reflection of his determination, dedication, and encouragement.

# Foreword

Dieting is an obsession for the American public. We all want to have our cake and eat it, too. Food is one of the great pleasures of life, and dieting is no fun. But when one of every two Americans is overweight, obviously something isn't working.

While it's true that many of us are born with genes for conserving energy and hanging on to fat, I believe that the real reason so many Americans are overweight can be found in the lifestyles we choose to live. We eat foods largely based on taste, with little concern for the hidden fats and calories these foods carry, and we eat all the time. Soon you may be able to order snack foods at the gas pump while you're waiting for the tank to fill up. While your car will burn all the gasoline going into the gas tank, you probably won't burn all the snack-food calories you're pouring into your body. It's hard to go into a fast-food restaurant and get out eating less than 800 to 1,000 calories worth of high-fat foods. So it takes very little effort to stay overweight, and lots of effort to fight off the temptation to eat great-tasting, high-fat foods.

In my practice, about 80 percent of the patients are women. This book is written by women for women everywhere, as well as for their husbands and families. Why is there such a preponderance of women complaining about weight gain? The answer almost certainly lies in two areas: physiology and cultural evolution. On the physiological side, body fat is a secondary sex characteristic of women. Fat in the hips and thighs accumulates after puberty, and at any given height and weight women have more fat as a percentage of body weight than men of the same height and weight. Desirable body fat percentages in women range between 22 and 28 percent, while in men they range between 15 and 20 percent.

For many adult women, fat accumulation begins with postpregnancy weight gain. During pregnancy, hormones produced by the placenta increase appetite and promote fat deposition. These fat stores were intended by nature to provide calories for breast-milk production in the postnatal period. Most ancient cultures practice breastfeeding for a year after a child is born, and during this time breast milk removes about 500 calories per day from the body, leading to a loss of the fat accumulated during pregnancy. However, American women often nurse their babies for a shorter period of time and often increase their food intake during breastfeeding, so that postpregnancy weight gain is not reversed. As a woman reaches her fifties and the approach of menopause, there is also a decrease in muscle mass. This loss of muscle leads to a decrease in metabolic rate, so that even with constant food intake there is some weight gain. There is also a redistribution of body fat into the upper body. Women who continue to eat the same amounts of food they always have find that with decreasing energy expenditure they gain weight that they feel they cannot lose.

To further aggravate the problem, the ideal of the attractive woman has changed. Today, the average female model is about five feet nine inches tall and about 110 pounds, while the average American woman is about five feet four inches tall and 125 pounds. This discrepancy can put pressure on women to achieve an unrealistic and sometimes unhealthy body weight.

While many diets are based on the idea that fat, protein, or carbohydrates contain some magic property to be exploited or avoided, it's crucial to understand that the human body can convert calories from protein to fat, from fat to carbohydrates, and back again. This means that anything you eat—from a cheesecake to a sandwich to a steak—can turn into body fat if it isn't burned as fuel. The reasons some diets work and others don't can't be found in a simplistic biochemical statement about eating any specific food type in any specific amount.

Of course, there are differences among individuals. I have known patients who would be able to lose weight easily and get away with pretty poor eating habits. On the other hand, I have had patients who eat very well and cannot lose weight easily. But losing weight with ease or with difficulty has nothing to do with counting proteins or carbs or fat grams. Humankind has had to survive on different diets in different climates, and so there are no simple weight-loss guidelines in terms of the three basic types of foods.

The idea that we can achieve weight loss by using meal-replacement shakes or bars may seem magical, but it's not. A Slim•Fast meal replacement takes the place of a meal, while providing a balance of nutrients designed to help you lose weight. For example, consider what happens when you try a meal replacement instead of a deli-counter tuna sandwich for lunch: the tuna sandwich would have 722 calories, 54 grams of fat, and only some of the essential vitamins and minerals you need every day. The meal replacement, on the other hand, has 220 calories, 3 grams of fat, and up to one-third of the daily requirement for vitamins and minerals. For calcium, which is important for strong bones, it contains up to 40 percent of the daily requirement in a single serving. In addition to starting the day with a delicious Slim•Fast shake, I suggest to my patients that they keep a six-pack of canned shakes in the car in case they miss a meal. It beats pulling into a fast-food restaurant on the way home.

A meal replacement is not meant to be your only source of nutrition. It is not intended to replace all of your eating in any day. It is meant to replace one or two meals each day and perhaps some snacks. When you're losing weight using meal replacements you eat fewer calories and fat, and you get more nutrition. Each meal replacement shake or bar contains many of the carbohydrates, protein, fiber, calcium, and other vitamins and minerals you need.

The basic truth none of us can avoid is this: In order to lose weight you must take in fewer calories than you are burning. Unfortunately, if you try to do this by just eating less, you will miss out on many of the important nutrients you need. You may get too little protein or too little calcium. By learning to use meal replacements as part of an overall lifestyle makeover, you'll cut calories while still getting healthy nutrition in a program that will help you keep these new habits going for a lifetime. You'll find great ways to exercise and increase everyday physical activity. Most of all, you'll be able to tailor this approach to fit your personal lifestyle.

As a physician who has helped people lose weight for over twenty years,

I know that it is most important that you make this diet plan your own. This book will provide you with everything you need to know, but only you can do everything you need to do. As you start out on this adventure of personal evaluation, renewal, and makeover, I send along my best wishes for the best of health.

—David Heber, M.D., Ph.D.
Professor of Medicine and Public Health
Director, UCLA Center for Human Nutrition

# Preface

Twenty years ago, a friend introduced me to Danny Abraham and Dr. Ed Steinberg. They appeared in my apartment "after work"—at 11 P.M.—to quiz me, a nutritionist, about what it would take to develop a product that could serve as a low-calorie meal for people trying to lose weight. At that time, 800-calorie-a-day liquid diets administered under a physician's supervision were becoming very popular. Danny and Ed wanted to develop a good-tasting product that could be purchased over-the-counter and used safely by anyone wanting to lose weight. This led to the birth of the Slim•Fast shake.

Over subsequent years, at nearly every meeting we had, Danny and Ed asked me, "How would you best describe Slim•Fast?" To me, the answer was easy. The product was made from milk fortified with vitamins, minerals, and fiber, and contained no appetite suppressants or other weight-loss drugs. It was obviously a food. Slim•Fast is a meal replacement and falls within the category established by the United States Food and Drug Administration called "food for special dietary purposes."

The Slim•Fast Foods Company decided to branch out into a wide variety of foods with an emphasis on great taste and balanced nutrition. Danny and Ed wanted the Slim•Fast products to go beyond helping you lose weight: They wanted a product that would actually improve your health by providing the kind of balanced nutrition that you probably cannot get in your regular diet.

Still, the Slim•Fast products had to overcome the popularity of fad diets that emphasized one food (like grapefruit or rice) or one vitamin or mineral (like beta-carotene or chromium picolinate) that promised to melt away pounds magically. The Slim•Fast Plan had staying power that these fad diets didn't, and it sustained itself through numerous food and nutrition trends.

For instance, Slim•Fast remained popular when everyone was loading up on fat-free cookies, pasta, and other starchy carbohydrates, and remained just as strong when people turned to high-protein diets.

Now, more than two million people use Slim•Fast products every day. The Slim•Fast Foods Company prides itself on its quality products, which have helped thousands of individuals attain a more healthful body weight. More important, the products and programs have helped countless individuals maintain their newly acquired body weight and a healthful lifestyle.

The Slim•Fast Plan works. It is safe, healthful, convenient, economical, and clinically proven to take off weight and keep it off. The plan is easy to follow and allows you to eat several times a day. You replace two meals with a Slim•Fast shake or meal bar and eat a sensible dinner and nutritious snacks in between meals. In this way, you don't have to feel hungry and never feel too stuffed. Between the vegetables you get at dinner and the fruit as snacks, you'll get five to nine servings a day of fruits and vegetables, the amount recommended by the National Cancer Institute and the American Heart Association to help lower your risk of cancer and heart disease. The plan will also provide you with an added boost of energy, which will motivate you to exercise. Once you've lost the weight, you'll find that the plan can help you keep the weight off. Reducing your calorie intake by just 250 to 400 calories per day can enable you to maintain a substantial weight loss for life. That's one fewer dessert or one Slim•Fast meal replacement each day instead of your usual meal.

The Slim•Fast Foods Company's commitment to excellence is reflected in more than twenty scientific studies, some of which have been ongoing for more than six years and published in scientific journals. A fully staffed Slim•Fast Nutrition Institute, which has medical, regulatory, and research and development departments, helps sustain these worldwide studies.

More than 55 percent of the United States' adult population is overweight or obese. This epidemic, now growing throughout the world, is accompanied by a greater risk of early death, heart disease, stroke, diabetes, osteoarthritis, infertility, and certain cancers. In an effort to prevent the 300,000 deaths caused by obesity each year, the Slim•Fast Foods Company has joined in partnerships and alliances with such groups as the North American Association for the Study of Obesity, the American Society for Clinical Nutrition, and the Partnership for Healthy Weight Management, a coalition of government, public, and private groups.

As a current user of the Slim•Fast Plan, I had the occasion to appreciate how successful the plan has been for me when a friend, who first met me twenty-five years ago, recently told me, "You were heavier then." I've found that I experience less hunger and am reassured knowing that I'm getting a rich supply of the vitamins and nutrients I need through the Slim•Fast shakes.

Each day in the clinic where I work I am faced with the pain and suffering that results from the disease of obesity. I saw my beloved aunt die from obesity-related illnesses. At age seventy-five, my father succumbed to heart disease that resulted from a poor diet high in saturated fat and cholesterol. I am grateful that a solution exists that is flexible, delicious, and can be shared with three generations of my family members.

Many of us can look forward to living well past one hundred if we choose the right path—a path of sensible eating, plenty of exercise, and a healthy mind-set. This is the path that will keep you trim and fit and enable you to experience all the pleasures life has to offer.

—George Blackburn, M.D., Ph.D.
Associate Director of Nutrition and Associate Professor of Surgery,
Harvard Medical School,
Beth Israel Deaconess Medical Center

# Slim•Fast and I

Even when I was just beginning my career in the mid-1960s, I couldn't model anything I didn't believe in. On the very first Paris collection I ever shot for *Vogue* magazine, I was handed a leopard-skin coat—and handed it right back. I just couldn't put it on. It almost made me cry. This could easily have been the end of my career; you don't say no to *Vogue* when things are just getting started for you. I told the editor why I couldn't wear the coat and why I didn't think they should show it; she told the photographer; somebody called Diana Vreeland, *Vogue*'s poohbah, and not only did they drop the leopard coats (instead of me!) from their pages that year, but Vreeland also dropped a word at a Washington dinner soon thereafter, and the next thing you know, it was illegal to import wild spotted fur into America.

So I learned early on about influence. The day the surgeon general announced that smoking was harmful to one's health, I saw Irving Penn talking on the phone to his agent and forbidding him to take any cigarette accounts—giving up some serious money. A little while later a cigarette company asked me to do a giant campaign for them, offering more money than I'd ever been offered for a job until that time. I was still a smoker myself, but I said *absolutely not*—I may have been a user (back then), but I wasn't a pusher. I've always tried to take care with the associations I make, so I'll never have to look back later and wonder whether I may have harmed anyone.

When I first started hearing about Slim•Fast, I was skeptical. I'd spent my last thirty-six professional years as Ms. Natural. For ages I've tried to be careful about what I ate, and a lot of my family and friends are health-food devotees or vegetarians. One of my sisters has been organic-only since the 1960s, and her children have never even had anything cooked in animal or fish stock, much less actually eaten any meat. Serious vegans forever.

"You are what you eat" was one of the youthful slogans of my slogan-happy generation.

But the truth is that in recent years I hadn't been feeling as good about my body as I used to—and for good reason. Over a period of fifteen years, I'd put on 22 percent of my original body weight—going from 115 to 140 pounds. When I realized that, I knew I had to make a change in my lifestyle. The average American puts on a pound a year after the age of twenty-one; after I turned forty, I found I was putting that on all at once. When I was home I'd eat right, but too often I found myself on the run, eating my way through room-service menus at the nicer hotels and grabbing fast food when I was staying at small-town Holiday Inns. I've done a lot of movies, and when you're on a location shoot you often spend ten hours a day waiting and only a few working; when you're waiting that long, one of the few things you have to look forward to is food, and sometimes I'd order more than I should, just hoping I'd find something that tasted good.

After all, I was young and as slim as I'd ever be; I didn't have to watch my weight . . . or so I thought, until I woke up one day 25 pounds heavier than I'd ever been. Once I turned forty, my body no longer felt the way it always had; all at once it felt uncomfortable, like a heavy, ill-fitting suit of clothes. I'd never felt my thighs rubbing together, but there they were! Suddenly my upper arms were brushing against my sides—at first I didn't even know what that feeling was. At work I started standing sideways to look thinner—it was amazing that I managed to fake my way through modeling as long as I did.

And it wasn't just the weight that bothered me; I just didn't have the energy I used to. At around this time I also attended a medical program to help me quit smoking (more on that later), which taught me a lot about health but left me more concerned than ever about the state of my body. I tried for years to take off the weight, but I hated the idea of a diet—I couldn't even stand to use the word. But I knew had to do something.

That's when I first started thinking about trying a program like Slim•Fast. Of course, not everyone had an open mind when I broached the subject with them. Many of my friends—including the ones who'd known me the longest—couldn't believe what I was saying. *But Slim•Fast comes in a can!*, they said. And I have to admit that I had my doubts, too. It sounded like Madison Avenue funny business to me, like the kind of quick-fix gimmick my generation had always been taught to resist.

But then something happened that really got my attention, and it involved one of my favorite things to do in life—scuba diving.

Ever since one brilliant day in Cozumel, Mexico, in 1965, when I first walked into the sea wearing a scuba tank, I've been a fanatic about diving. For about fifteen years after that I dove all over the world, whenever I had the chance, until my once-stable personal life began getting the bends and scuba diving became less of a priority. But in recent years I'd really begun to miss it, and in 1997 I finally got started again when I headed for the wreck diver's Valhalla—the Truk Lagoon in Micronesia, where during World War II American bombers sunk more than forty Japanese munitions boats and shot down more than thirty Zero fighter planes. Half a century later they're still there, 60 to 180 feet below the surface; covered in masses of soft coral in bright red, orange, and yellow, they look like the product of a summit meeting between Michelangelo and Walt Disney. The diving there is unbeatable, and my love affair with diving was rekindled immediately.

Diving is exhilarating; taking the plunge into that lagoon is like falling backward into Botticelli's clamshell, arms outstretched—Venus laughing. But it's also tough business. When you're scurrying around more than a hundred feet below the surface, you're often subject to vicious currents—and when a thick wave of silt is stirred up in the atmosphere around you, it can be difficult to find the way out. That's why I was so glad to meet my true dive buddies when I started diving seriously again—a bunch of world-class divers who make a living out of all this adventure. Mitch Scaggs, Tanya Burnett, Brett Gillum, and Dan Ruth: These are the bad boys (and girl) who allow me to join their underwater team whenever I'm in their neck of the woods—which is anywhere in the world.

Whenever I get a new idea, I have a habit of polling my closest friends, the ones who know me best, to see whether they think it makes sense. So when I began thinking about trying Slim•Fast, I mentioned it to my diving pals. I didn't know what to expect; this is a pretty macho bunch, after all. But I sure didn't expect the response I got: they'd *all* used Slim•Fast themselves, and they loved it. Dan had lost 50 pounds on it, and he returns to it whenever his wetsuit gets a little tight. These professional divers are some pretty tough characters; they face danger every day and come up laughing. If *they* were Slim•Fast regulars, that told me one thing—those shakes obviously aren't for sissies.

So I started looking into Slim•Fast a little more deeply. I knew that what I needed was a way to get a calorie-controlled, nutritionally balanced diet every day, and I knew myself well enough to know that following it had better be *easy*. And what I learned is that the Slim•Fast Plan is no gimmick. It's a program, designed by leading nutritionists and proven in decades of studies and consumer success stories, that helps you to achieve a balanced diet every day—to get your full complement of vitamins and nutrients, all wrapped up in two shakes (or meal bars) a day and a sensible dinner. There's even an allowance for snacks on the side. With up to twenty-four vitamins and minerals going for it, it's a much healthier regimen than most of us consume every day—certainly better than I was eating. And so I decided to try it.

The results? I loved the taste of the Creamy Milk Chocolate Slim•Fast shake immediately; it tasted like the chocolate milk of my childhood. So I knew I could make Slim•Fast part of my life. There were no schedules to follow, no elaborate meals to prepare. It was versatile; if I knew I had to have a big business lunch, I could have a shake for breakfast and another one for dinner— and that in turn gave me more time to do other things, like sneaking in a little exercise or doing some reading.

And here's a thing you should know: It didn't all happen at once. Nothing's perfect in this world, and when I started off with Slim•Fast I didn't fully commit right away—I'd have a shake here and there but then get distracted by some appealing meal and fall off. But after a week or two I found myself sticking to the program full-time—two shakes a day, a sensible meal, and some moderate exercise. And the most important thing was the simplest: It worked. I began losing weight, and feeling wonderful and energetic at the same time. By the time three weeks had passed I'd lost 7 pounds; a few weeks later I was down 12. At the age of fifty-six, I now weigh 129 pounds for the first time since I was . . . thirty-six? Forty-one? I can't even remember. And I'm still losing! The other day I tried on a sleek red dress I've had for years—a real beauty that hasn't fit me in ages—and it slipped right on! There's no other way to put it: I feel terrific.

And that's why I was happy about doing this book. The people at Slim•Fast have been helping folks lose weight and get healthy for decades; by now there are millions of us successful dieters using their shakes and bars on a regular basis. But the Slim•Fast team knows that staying healthy for life is about more than just dropping a few pounds—too many crash dieters have tried that quick-fix approach, and then put the weight right back on as soon as they got tired of eating grapefruit or steak and eggs all day. When I first began meeting with Slim•Fast's medical experts, what really impressed me was their broader message: Losing weight is a choice anyone can make. All it takes is a few minor adjustments in lifestyle: Start eating right. Find some exercises you enjoy. Take a few steps to reduce stress in your life. And before you know it, the Slim•Fast Plan will have you looking better and feeling fantastic. We call it the Slim•Fast Body•Mind•Life Makeover.

All Debbie Kotz and I have tried to do in this book is show you how to get your own makeover started. Along the way you'll hear from plenty of people like me who've been through just what you're going through now: Remember, you can be one of the millions who are doing this successfully. Whether it's 7 pounds or 75 pounds you have to lose, all it takes is a little change in your eating habits, and they'll change before you know it. Once you're under way, I'll bet you'll find it as easy as I have to get fit and remake your life.

Get started! You'll be a new you before you know it. I know I am. And I'm rooting for you.

# 1

# CHANGE YOUR BODY, CHANGE YOUR LIFE

**H**ow many times have you stared at yourself in the mirror and thought, "If only . . ." If only I could be trimmer, fitter, healthier . . . If only I could button up my old jeans . . . Someday—maybe next September, next April, next summer, next year . . . If only I could find a way to remake my life . . .

When it comes to your body, you've probably spent a lot of time on this kind of wishful thinking. But the very fact that you're opening this book means you're ready to consider turning your "if only's" into positive and lasting action.

Perhaps you've been overweight all your life, or perhaps, like many people, you've gone from fat to thin and back again. Or maybe you've only recently realized that the one, two, or three pounds you've been gaining every year have really added up.

Well, no matter what your circumstances, there's no time like the present to change your life. With the Slim•Fast Body•Mind•Life Makeover, losing weight—and keeping it off for life—can be within your grasp. It's a plan that has been tested in universities and proven in households all over the world: Through a combination of balanced nutrition, exercise, and other beneficial changes in your way of living, you can have the body you want . . . and the life you deserve.

If your weight is weighing heavily on your mind, you're certainly not alone. Losing weight is an obsession in our culture. Despite the fact that more than 50 percent of Americans are overweight, we're bombarded with images of impossibly slender actresses and models splashed across TV screens and the covers of countless magazines. What we don't see is their nonstop and often very unhealthy dieting.

In an effort to attain that kind of "ideal" body, many of us have turned to sporadic dieting—only to be sorely disappointed in the end. For at least twenty-five years, we've been searching in frustration for a quick-fix way to lose weight, in an attempt to trick our bodies into shedding those extra pounds. We earnestly believed that all-protein diets would keep us thin for life. Once we gained the weight back after going off those diets, we turned to the grapefruit diet, then the food-combining diet (eating certain foods at certain times of the day), and before we knew it we were back on the high-protein kick. But who wants to live under rigid eating rules for a lifetime? When the restrictions got too taxing, we dropped the diets and went back to our old eating habits.

No wonder we're fed up with trying to lose weight. Who can blame you if your first thought when hearing about a new weight-loss product or plan is: *What's the catch?*

Well, your instincts are right. Most such products and plans do have a catch: They're all temporary ways to take off weight, and none can ever promise that you'll stay thin forever. That's because when you buy into one of these gimmicks, you're buying into the notion that you're going on a diet just long enough to lose weight. Once you've gone through boot camp and lost the weight, you're led to believe that you can go AWOL and abandon any of the restrictions you were following.

You've probably heard this before, or experienced it firsthand: Losing weight isn't the hardest part—it's keeping the pounds off that's tricky. Any yo-yo dieter can attest to this fact, and dieting statistics confirm it. As many as 75 to 90 percent of people who lose weight eventually gain back the weight they've lost, and sometimes they gain even more.

The leading obesity experts now realize that most dieters haven't figured out what it takes to maintain weight loss—and that most weight-loss programs don't really teach people to make the changes they'll need to keep the pounds off for life. Many such programs focus on getting you to your goal weight without giving you the tools for staying there. The drastic behavior changes most require to lose weight—from attending weekly sessions to restricting your diet to unpalatable foods—are usually too severe to stay on forever.

In order to beat the odds and be a successful dieter, you need to make small, simple changes that you can fold naturally into your lifestyle—to give yourself that one-two punch that will allow you to lose the weight you want *and* keep it off for life.

This book is designed to help you do just that. The plan it offers, designed and refined by a team of nutritionists over more than two decades, can help you lose weight sensibly so you can live a long, healthy life. It will help you make over not only your body, but your mind and your life. And here's the best thing about it: Simple and easy to follow, this plan can actually enable you to enjoy your life more than ever before. Once you start losing weight, you'll likely start feeling better, experience a greater sense of energy, have more self-confidence, and exult in the knowledge that you've taken your health in your own hands.

The makeover is based on the proven Slim•Fast Plan that has helped countless dieters remake their bodies and transform their lives. Convenient, inexpensive, proven in years of medical trials, the Slim•Fast Plan has long been established as one of the healthiest and most dependable ways to lose weight. Over the years, many of these successful dieters have written to the makers of Slim•Fast to describe how easily the plan fit their lifestyles. One dieter, Michele Kemlar of Beverly Hills, California, echoes the experience of countless others: "A year ago," she writes,

I was feeling very upset about my weight, which was 212 pounds at the time. I'm a private-duty nurse and was employed at the time caring for a newborn (and you know how busy that can be). Breakfast and lunch, the smaller meals, were easier to prepare, but I found it hard to prepare a proper dinner for myself because the baby needed so much attention; I wasn't eating right. I'd heard from friends how convenient and delicious Slim•Fast was, so I decided to give it a try. My energy level soared, and I lost over 80 pounds in ten months! I went from 212 pounds to under 132; my dress size went from a 22–24 to a 6–8. And I feel great! I've yo-yo dieted all my life, but this is the first time since junior high school that I've seen this weight!

Give yourself the Slim•Fast Body•Mind•Life Makeover, and you may well find yourself as fit and energized as Michele. By making over your body, you'll find yourself growing toned and fit as you cut your calorie intake and burn fat through exercise. By making over your mind, you'll reduce the stress in your life and experience the renewed self-esteem that comes with losing weight, exercising, and improving your health. By making over your life, you'll find you're happier with yourself on every level—from the way you look to the way you feel about yourself. And from that, changes can follow in all parts of your life.

## Is Your Weight in the Danger Zone?

While you're weighing your decision about whether to embark on a journey to a new weight and a new life, you might want to consider the health implications of being overweight. You probably already know that obesity can lead to a host of health problems, from heart disease to diabetes. But how much is too much? If you're otherwise healthy, what's the harm in carrying an extra forty pounds? Plenty, according to the latest research. Being even moderately overweight carries certain health risks, and being obese is downright dangerous; one new study found that obese people have a two-and-a-half-times-greater chance of dying from weight-related illnesses than those who are only somewhat overweight.

The best way to judge whether your weight is endangering your own health is by calculating your body mass index (BMI). This is a scientific formula that uses your height and weight to create an index of just how healthy your weight is; researchers use BMI measurements when studying the prevalence of disease in overweight and obese populations. To calculate your BMI, simply plug your height and weight into the chart on the following page. A BMI below 25 means you're at low risk for disease; 25 to 29 puts you at moderately increased risk, and if your BMI is 30 or above, you're at the highest risk.

Your BMI may not sound like good news, but as you lose weight you'll

# Body Mass Index Chart

## Height (Feet and Inches)

| Weight (Pounds) | 5'0" | 5'1" | 5'2" | 5'3" | 5'4" | 5'5" | 5'6" | 5'7" | 5'8" | 5'9" | 5'10" | 5'11" | 6'0" | 6'1" | 6'2" | 6'3" | 6'4" |
|---|---|---|---|---|---|---|---|---|---|---|---|---|---|---|---|---|---|
| 100 | 20 | 19 | 18 | 18 | 17 | 17 | 16 | 16 | 15 | 15 | 14 | 14 | 14 | 13 | 13 | 12 | 12 |
| 105 | 21 | 20 | 19 | 19 | 18 | 17 | 17 | 16 | 16 | 16 | 15 | 15 | 14 | 14 | 13 | 13 | 13 |
| 110 | 21 | 21 | 20 | 19 | 19 | 18 | 18 | 17 | 17 | 16 | 16 | 15 | 15 | 15 | 14 | 14 | 13 |
| 115 | 22 | 22 | 21 | 20 | 20 | 19 | 19 | 18 | 17 | 17 | 17 | 16 | 16 | 15 | 15 | 14 | 14 |
| 120 | 23 | 23 | 22 | 21 | 21 | 20 | 19 | 19 | 18 | 18 | 17 | 17 | 16 | 16 | 15 | 15 | 15 |
| 125 | 24 | 24 | 23 | 22 | 21 | 21 | 20 | 20 | 19 | 18 | 18 | 17 | 17 | 16 | 16 | 16 | 15 |
| 130 | 25 | 25 | 24 | 23 | 22 | 22 | 21 | 20 | 20 | 19 | 19 | 18 | 18 | 17 | 17 | 16 | 16 |
| 135 | 26 | 26 | 25 | 24 | 23 | 22 | 22 | 21 | 21 | 20 | 19 | 19 | 18 | 18 | 17 | 17 | 16 |
| 140 | 27 | 26 | 26 | 25 | 24 | 23 | 23 | 22 | 21 | 21 | 20 | 20 | 19 | 18 | 18 | 17 | 17 |
| 145 | 28 | 27 | 27 | 26 | 25 | 24 | 23 | 23 | 22 | 21 | 21 | 20 | 20 | 19 | 19 | 18 | 18 |
| 150 | 29 | 28 | 27 | 27 | 26 | 25 | 24 | 23 | 23 | 22 | 22 | 21 | 20 | 20 | 19 | 19 | 18 |
| 155 | 30 | 29 | 28 | 27 | 27 | 26 | 25 | 24 | 24 | 23 | 22 | 22 | 21 | 20 | 20 | 19 | 19 |
| 160 | 31 | 30 | 29 | 28 | 27 | 27 | 26 | 25 | 24 | 24 | 23 | 22 | 22 | 21 | 21 | 20 | 19 |
| 165 | 32 | 31 | 30 | 29 | 28 | 27 | 27 | 26 | 25 | 24 | 24 | 23 | 22 | 22 | 21 | 21 | 20 |
| 170 | 33 | 32 | 31 | 30 | 29 | 28 | 27 | 27 | 26 | 25 | 24 | 24 | 23 | 22 | 22 | 21 | 21 |
| 175 | 34 | 33 | 32 | 31 | 30 | 29 | 28 | 27 | 27 | 26 | 25 | 24 | 24 | 23 | 22 | 22 | 21 |
| 180 | 35 | 34 | 33 | 32 | 31 | 30 | 29 | 28 | 27 | 27 | 26 | 25 | 24 | 24 | 23 | 22 | 22 |
| 185 | 36 | 35 | 34 | 33 | 32 | 31 | 30 | 29 | 28 | 27 | 27 | 26 | 25 | 24 | 24 | 23 | 23 |
| 190 | 37 | 36 | 35 | 34 | 33 | 32 | 31 | 30 | 29 | 28 | 27 | 26 | 26 | 25 | 24 | 24 | 23 |
| 195 | 38 | 37 | 36 | 35 | 33 | 32 | 31 | 31 | 30 | 29 | 28 | 27 | 26 | 26 | 25 | 24 | 24 |
| 200 | 39 | 38 | 37 | 35 | 34 | 33 | 32 | 31 | 30 | 30 | 29 | 28 | 27 | 26 | 26 | 25 | 24 |
| 205 | 40 | 39 | 37 | 36 | 35 | 34 | 33 | 32 | 31 | 30 | 29 | 29 | 28 | 27 | 26 | 26 | 25 |
| 210 | 41 | 40 | 38 | 37 | 36 | 35 | 34 | 33 | 32 | 31 | 30 | 29 | 28 | 28 | 27 | 26 | 26 |
| 215 | 42 | 41 | 39 | 38 | 37 | 36 | 35 | 34 | 33 | 32 | 31 | 30 | 29 | 28 | 28 | 27 | 26 |
| 220 | 43 | 42 | 40 | 39 | 38 | 37 | 36 | 34 | 33 | 32 | 32 | 31 | 30 | 29 | 28 | 27 | 27 |
| 225 | 44 | 43 | 41 | 40 | 39 | 37 | 36 | 35 | 34 | 33 | 32 | 31 | 31 | 30 | 29 | 28 | 27 |
| 230 | 45 | 43 | 42 | 41 | 39 | 38 | 37 | 36 | 35 | 34 | 33 | 32 | 31 | 30 | 30 | 29 | 28 |
| 235 | 46 | 44 | 43 | 42 | 40 | 39 | 38 | 37 | 36 | 35 | 34 | 33 | 32 | 31 | 30 | 29 | 29 |
| 240 | 47 | 45 | 44 | 43 | 41 | 40 | 39 | 38 | 36 | 35 | 34 | 33 | 33 | 32 | 31 | 30 | 29 |
| 245 | 48 | 46 | 45 | 43 | 42 | 41 | 40 | 38 | 37 | 36 | 35 | 34 | 33 | 32 | 31 | 31 | 30 |
| 250 | 49 | 47 | 46 | 44 | 43 | 42 | 40 | 39 | 38 | 37 | 36 | 35 | 34 | 33 | 32 | 31 | 30 |

☐ Underweight  ☐ Weight Appropriate  ☐ Overweight  ☐ Obese

find that the chart can give you incentive to continue: As you progress with the makeover, check back with this chart and you'll be able to watch, week by week, as your health steadily improves.

Determining your BMI will also reveal just how high your risk is for developing certain health conditions. The following findings are based on a 1998 report issued by the National Heart, Lung and Blood Institute on the health hazards of being overweight. This is crucial information, demonstrating that losing weight is important not just to help you look better, but to help you avoid serious health risks. Consider this all as good news: Losing excess pounds can actually help you avoid many of the greatest risks to your health.

**Hypertension**: Your risk of high blood pressure increases with every excess pound you carry. If you have a BMI of 30 or greater, you have a 38 percent risk of developing high blood pressure if you're a man and 32 percent if you're a woman; men and women whose BMI is under 30, in contrast, have only an 18 percent and 17 percent chance, respectively.

**High cholesterol**: Higher body weight is directly associated with high cholesterol levels. Your levels of HDL ("good" cholesterol) drop as you gain weight, while your LDL ("bad" cholesterol) and triglycerides (which should never rise above moderate levels) rise. If you carry more fat around your abdomen (compared to your hips), you may also be at higher risk for having high cholesterol.

**Diabetes**: Recent studies have found that gaining just 11 pounds or more after age eighteen increases your risk of developing Type 2 diabetes. Specifically, your risk of diabetes increases by about 25 percent for every 1 unit increase in your BMI above 22.

**Heart disease**: Your risk of suffering a heart attack or developing heart disease increases even with modest increases in your weight. In the Nurses' Health Study, researchers found that moderately overweight women (with BMIs of 25 to 28) had twice the risk of developing heart disease and that obese women (with BMIs of 29 or greater) had three times the risk compared to women who weren't overweight.

**Stroke**: Recent studies have shown that your risk of suffering a stroke increases with your weight. If your BMI is greater than 27, you have a 75 percent higher risk of suffering a stroke; if it's greater than 32, you have a 137 percent higher risk compared to slender women, according to one study published in the *Journal of the American Medical Association.*

**Arthritis**: People who carry around excess weight, not surprisingly, are far more likely to develop knee pain caused by arthritis. One recent study tracked sets of middle-aged female twins in which one twin had developed arthritis; the arthritic twins were on average about 7 to 11 pounds heavier than their sisters. The researchers estimated that for every 2- to 3-pound increase in weight (one BMI unit), an overweight woman's risk of developing arthritis increases by 9 to 13 percent. By the same token, a decrease in weight of two BMI units or more decreases the odds of developing arthritis in the knee by 50 percent.

**Cancer**: Being overweight has been linked directly with various forms of cancer. For example, if you are a woman with a BMI of 29 or more, you have twice the risk of developing colon cancer as a woman with a BMI of less than 21. If you tend to have more fat around your abdomen than around your hips, you have a higher risk of developing colon polyps, which can be precursors to cancer. Likewise, studies have shown that being obese increases your risk of dying from postmenopausal breast cancer; gaining just 20 pounds from age eighteen to midlife doubles your risk of breast cancer. And women with a BMI of 30 or more have three times more risk of developing endometrial cancer (cancer of the uterine lining) than a woman who is not overweight.

Here's a little trick you may find instructive: Figure out how much you're over your ideal weight. Divide that figure in two. Then fill two knapsacks with that amount of weight—in books, dumbbells, what have you, and carry them around with you all day. Once you take them off at night, you'll see what a relief it will be to lose the weight you should.

## Restoring Balance to Your Body and Life

As you're probably beginning to realize, you can put yourself in the driver's seat when it comes to improving your health. When you make the decision to replace your old eating habits with a new, healthy lifestyle, what you're doing is taking charge of your future. You're taking the necessary steps to restore the balance that's missing from your body and life.

Imagine for a moment that you're living a different life. You eat moderate amounts of food throughout the day, so you never get too hungry and never feel too stuffed. You give your body a wide variety of nutrients in the perfect amounts to keep you healthy, fit, and energized. You exercise your heart and muscles and work to improve your flexibility. You've learned to take time out to relax; you feel better about yourself, and your happiness shows through every day in your dealings with others. You take pleasure in your fit new body, and revel in the fact that you're living a healthier life.

This is no fantasy. This can be your future, if you're ready to give yourself the Body•Mind•Life Makeover.

Bekki Ackley of Orlando, Florida, wrote a letter to Slim•Fast explaining how the program changed her life:

> I had been overweight for most of my adult life. My weight ranged from 170 pounds to 210 pounds. I tried everything from acupuncture to diet pills. I consulted weight-loss doctors and therapists. Nothing seemed to work! Pursuing an acting and singing career would not allow me to be this heavy. I was actually told by a casting agent to leave and not come back until I lost 60 pounds. I was ready to give up, until I saw a commercial advertising your product. Although I was reluctant, I wanted more than anything to get the weight off and start my career.
>
> Now, two years later, I am five feet nine inches and 128 pounds! I have an agent and sing the National Anthem professionally for the Orlando Magic. I owe my success to Slim•Fast. I am a brand-new person, in terms of both my looks and my health. My doctor recently told me that I'm the healthiest patient he has—not to mention what it has done for my self-esteem. I am on top of the world!

The Slim•Fast Body•Mind•Life Makeover can help you the way it helped Bekki, by showing you how to eat nutritiously and get the maximum pleasure from the food you eat—without overindulging. You'll learn how to fit exercise into your schedule (no matter how busy you are), and how to choose activities you enjoy, so you'll always be ready to go. And you'll learn how to relax and take a step back from life's little annoyances, helping you focus on achieving your goals. If you nurture your body *and* your mind, you'll reap the ultimate reward: the life you've always wanted.

## Taking Charge of Your Health—With Slim•Fast

In the fast-paced world you live in, you may not have much time to eat properly. If you're running late in the morning, you may skip breakfast. Feeling famished in the late morning, you might be tempted to grab a doughnut or muffin while on the run. Lunch might consist of one long snack session from afternoon until evening. Dinner might be the only time you sit down and have a real meal—probably thrown together with whatever ingredients you happen to have on hand. Whatever your eating habits, chances are you don't think too hard about what you put into your mouth. You certainly don't have a computer in your head calculating all the calories, fat, vitamins, minerals, and nutrients in every morsel you eat.

Unless you're carefully plotting out every meal to ensure that you're getting a properly balanced variety of foods and an ample supply of fruits and vegetables, you're probably lacking many of the essential nutrients your body needs. What's more, when you try to control the foods you eat, you're probably underestimating the number of calories you're really eating in any meal or snack. That's why the Slim•Fast Plan was created—to help people get the nutrition a body needs, while controlling the number of calories they consume.

At the core of the plan are the Slim•Fast shakes, snack bars, and meal bars—a line of food products that, when consumed on a regular basis, help you get the fuel your body needs. Unlike some other diet products, Slim•Fast contains no appetite suppressants, "fat burners," or other additives that claim to speed weight loss. The Slim•Fast meal replacements and snacks are pure food—protein, dietary fiber, a healthy measure of carbohydrates and fat, and up to twenty-four essential vitamins and minerals—more than most people get with three full meals a day, with far fewer calories. Just two shakes or meal bars per day provide you with most of the vitamins and minerals you need to stay healthy.

Unlike liquid diets, the Slim•Fast Plan combines these products with a sensible meal and three snacks, so you won't miss out on the hundreds of nutrients that are found only in fruits, vegetables, fish, and whole grains. Combining the shakes with the several daily servings of fruits and vegetables on the plan will enable you to get 20 to 35 grams of fiber each day, the amount recommended by the American Dietetic Association and the National Cancer Institute to lower your risk of colon cancer and heart disease. It will also keep you feeling full between meals, so you won't be as tempted to sneak those snacks in between.

Many people find that the plan not only helps keep them fit but also gives them the boost of energy that comes from exercising, eating light, and eating right. Take the case of Darlene Nischwitz, of Caufield, Ohio, who wrote about her mother's experience with Slim•Fast.

On May 30, 1999, my mom, Gerry Plowman, celebrated her ninety-fifth birthday. She has been a fan of Slim•Fast for years. Most days, she has a Slim•Fast for two meals, occasionally one. Her cardiologist heartily endorses Slim•Fast because he knows it contains great nutrition. Mom also rides an exercise bike an hour a day (in twenty-minute intervals) and drinks eight glasses of water a day religiously. We are all in wonder of her.

Of course, losing excess weight goes hand in hand with improving your health. And the Body•Mind•Life Makeover is designed to help you do both. To lose weight on the eating plan, you simply combine two Slim•Fast shakes or meal bars each day with a sensible meal and two or three snacks; then, to maintain your ideal weight once you've reached it, you can switch to one shake a day with two sensible meals and snacks. As you'll see in the chapters to come, each meal should contain a healthy serving of protein, a salad, several servings of vegetables, a light serving of starch, and some fruit for dessert. The result is a plan you can live with—and live healthier than ever.

The Slim•Fast Plan has been rigorously tested in clinical trials throughout the world. In one study involving a hundred participants, researchers at an obesity clinic found that Slim•Fast worked better at taking off weight than their subjects' usual diet of traditional foods. At the University of Ulm in

Germany, volunteers who used two Slim•Fast meal replacements with a sensible meal and snacks every day for twelve weeks lost an average of over 15 pounds. Those who simply tried to cut their intake to between 1,200 and 1,500 calories a day of regular food (by counting calories themselves) lost only 3 pounds.

In a larger study conducted by David Heber, M.D., Ph.D., director of the UCLA Center for Human Nutrition, 300 participants followed the Slim•Fast Plan for twelve weeks to lose weight and then continued to use Slim•Fast for two years to maintain their weight loss. Of those who started, 91 percent completed the first twelve weeks for weight loss; among them, men lost an average of 19 pounds, women an average of 14. Three-quarters of the subjects continued the weight-maintenance part of the study. After two years, 51 percent of those participants stayed with the program: the men maintained an average weight loss of 14 pounds, the women 13.6.

So just following the Slim•Fast eating guidelines alone is a proven way to help you lose weight and maintain the loss for life. And yet there's so much more to the Body•Mind•Life Makeover than just eating right. By following the exercise and relaxation components of the plan as outlined in these pages, you'll find ways to boost your health and fitness even further—giving yourself every advantage in the great fitness challenge.

## Making the Exercise Connection

Until the latter half of the twentieth century, few people had to worry about getting enough exercise. They moved all day long without even thinking about it, walking to and from work, hauling their bags home from errands, and doing the fix-it jobs around the house themselves. In the car-driven, remote-control, and keyboard world in which we now live, we actually have to *work* to lead an active lifestyle. We schedule in exercise by joining gyms, hiring personal trainers, and buying the latest workout videos. Still, most of us quit our exercise programs within six months after we start.

Why is it so hard to make exercise part of our lives? The same reason it's so difficult to exercise successfully: We treat both diet and exercise as a means to an end. If we work out hard enough, we tell ourselves, we'll have the body we want. Trouble is, most of us can't possibly work out hard enough to attain the super-sleek figures we see on TV. (Most of those models are born with those bodies—or their managers force them to work out two or three hours a day to achieve them!) When we don't see the results we want right away, most of us get frustrated and quit. And let's face it: Exercise can seem like a chore—something to get out of the way before we can kick back and have fun. It's the easiest thing in the world to put off, the hardest regimen to stick with.

The exercise plan on the Body•Mind•Life Makeover challenges you to rethink your attitudes about exercise. It offers a wide variety of exercise options, as well as strategies to help you squeeze in activity throughout your day. The one requirement is that you choose an activity that you actually *enjoy,* and stick to it. Maybe you get a rush in-line skating through the park; maybe biking is more your speed, or hiking, or swimming. If you're having fun and feel energized after your workouts, you won't even think about quitting. After all, how many of us have trouble getting ourselves roused to hit the beach in the summer, or heading off on a long walk while we're on vacation? If you can find a few fun things you enjoy doing on a regular basis, get in the habit of doing them regularly and actively, and soon you'll find that exercise has become a part of your life you just can't live without.

The exercise component of the Body•Mind•Life Makeover calls for you to shift your body into active mode for one hour every day. Now, a full hour may sound like a lot, but if you break it down into smaller chunks—a fifteen-minute walk here, half an hour of biking after work—you should find it more than manageable. You'll also be breaking your workouts down into three different fitness areas: flexibility (stretches), strength (resistance training), and cardiovascular (steady movement like running, walking, and swimming). This combination will help you achieve a healthy, fit body. You'll shed fat and put on muscle, which will turn your body into a calorie-burning machine. You'll soon see that the exercise plan works hand in hand with the Slim•Fast eating plan to help maximize your weight-loss efforts. You'll also experience these other amazing health benefits:

**You'll be able to shed fat more easily.** The combination of steady exercise and strength training delivers a one-two punch to your fat cells: Steady exercise burns off excess calories, which can mobilize your fat cells to release fat, while at the same time a serious workout will elevate your metabolism for several hours after a workout, helping suppress your appetite temporarily. Strength training builds up muscle cells, which use more energy than fat cells, retraining your body to burn calories more quickly and efficiently—that is, triggering your body's natural weight-loss mechanism.

**You'll be happier with your body.** A study from Brigham Young University in Utah found that sedentary women who participated in a resistance training program for twelve weeks experienced an improved body image and improved self-esteem—even if they didn't lose any weight. The researchers concluded that the tangible results, from increased muscle definition to the amount of weight one can lift, helped participants recognize their progress.

**You'll have an easier time keeping the weight off.** A study of 150 people conducted by Kaiser Permanente in northern California found that 90 percent of those who maintained weight loss months after losing weight were exercising at least three times a week for thirty minutes or more; only 34 percent of those who regained their weight, on the other hand, were steady exercisers.

**You can turn back the clock and reverse some signs of aging.** Stretching can help counteract the loss of flexibility that occurs as the aging process begins to shorten your muscle fibers and tendons. As your body begins to be able to move more freely, you'll be helping yourself avoid lower-back and knee injuries, which occur more commonly as you get older. Strength training can also help you turn back the clock: One study found that elderly people who worked out with weights were able to increase their muscle mass at the same rate as twenty-five-year-olds on the same weight-training regimen. Another recent study from the University of Illinois at Urbana-Champaign found that previously sedentary people over age sixty who walked rapidly three days a week for forty-five minutes showed significant improvement in the mental abilities that otherwise decline with age.

# Taking a Daily Relaxation Vacation

How many times have you dug into a pint of rocky road ice cream to soothe you when you're stressed? How many times has a chocolate bar served as a little "pick-me-up" when you're feeling blue? All too often, you may turn to food when you're really not that hungry. Maybe you've had a particularly tense day, or you just can't lift yourself out of that slump. Maybe you're just feeling bored and need a dose of instant pleasure.

For years, researchers have been studying the link between food and mood. Researcher Judith Wurtman, Ph.D., of the Massachusetts Institute of Technology found that pretzels, cookies, and other starchy carbohydrates boost the feel-good brain chemical serotonin; she believes this may explain why women who suffer from premenstrual mood swings crave these snack foods. Other research indicates that chocolate can have mood-enhancing effects because it contains chemicals called cannabinoids—the same class of chemicals that produces a marijuana high. Regardless of whether your food cravings are biochemical or based on habits you learned as a child (like getting a chocolate chip cookie to soothe a scraped knee), they could be a stumbling block on your road to weight loss. The truth is, when you feel your spirits are flagging, a burst of nutritional energy—the kind you can get from a Slim•Fast snack bar—is a far better idea.

The Body•Mind•Life Makeover will teach you how to deal with life's little blahs and stresses without turning to food. You'll set aside twenty minutes a day (just skip one of those time-killer sitcoms) to get your body into a state of total relaxation. Think of this as a mini-vacation you can take every single day, a pocket of time to take a break from your fast-paced world.

This plan works in concert with the eating and exercise plans to help you lose weight by managing stress in healthier ways. Like the exercise plan, the relaxation program offers a variety of techniques, allowing you to choose the one that works best for you. The aim is to feel refreshed after a long day, and renewed for the day you'll be facing tomorrow. You'll find yourself looking forward to your "away time" every day—that little slice of time when you can put away your cares and concentrate on your happiness.

This relaxation plan may sound a little New Age-y, but it's actually grounded in solid science. In over two decades of research, Herbert Benson, M.D., associate professor of medicine at Harvard Medical School and author of *The Relaxation Response*, has determined that relaxation can have a host of health benefits—from lowering your risk of heart disease to curing insomnia. Relaxation also lowers your body's production of stress hormones, which are thought to trigger food cravings by throwing your blood sugar levels out of balance. On the flip side, relaxation boosts your brain's production of the "happy" chemicals, serotonin and endorphins. In short, taking some time daily to relax can help you get the same mellow, pleasurable feeling you may be accustomed to getting from a big piece of chocolate cake. And wouldn't you feel better knowing that you're relaxing *and* helping remake your body, all at once?

## Setting Your Weight-Loss Goal

Before you can embark on a weight-loss program, you need to figure out how much weight you want to lose. This can be pretty tricky, considering that the more weight you lose, the greater the chance that you'll gain it all back. This may seem like a cruel trick of nature, but it's actually common sense: The less you weigh, the fewer calories your body needs to maintain your new weight. In other words, if you go from 180 pounds down to 120, your body—which needed 2,700 calories per day to maintain your heavier weight—will now need only 1,800. That's a whopping 900 calories a day difference between your old and your new eating habits—the equivalent of a hefty lunch in a restaurant. On the other hand, if you go from 180 pounds to 150, your body will need only 450 fewer calories each day to maintain your weight—a cutback most people should be able to achieve simply by keeping an eye on their portions.

Remember: Losing the weight is only half the battle. Maintaining the loss is what wins the war.

**Write down your weight-loss goal:**                    _____

The rate at which you'll lose weight will vary depending on how much you currently weigh. The Slim•Fast eating plan contains 1,400 to 1,500 calories per day—about 1,000 calories fewer than many people normally eat. If you normally consume 1,900 calories a day, for example, you can lose a pound a week by going on the plan—cutting your intake by 500 calories each day, or 3,500 calories per seven-day week.

There's an easy formula to help you determine your current calorie intake: simply multiply your body weight (in pounds) by the number 15.

Here are a couple of examples:

> 180-pound woman
> 180 lbs x 15 = 2,700
>                        −1,000
> Calorie intake:    1,700 to lose 2 pounds a week

On the 1,400- to 1,500-calorie eating plan, she would lose two and a half pounds per week for the first few weeks. Her rate of weight loss would then gradually slow down as she continued to lose weight and her body required fewer and fewer calories.

> 200-pound man
> 200 lbs x 15 = 3,000
>                        −1,000
> Calorie intake:    2,000 to lose 2 pounds a week

On the 1,400- to-1,500-calorie-a-day eating plan, he would lose 4 to 5 pounds per week for the first few weeks, then lose at a declining rate as his body required fewer and fewer calories to maintain his lower weight.

**Write down your current calorie intake:** _____

**Estimate how quickly you should be**
   **losing weight on the plan:** _____

   (Note: The ideal rate of weight loss is 1 to 2 pounds per week. If you are losing weight much faster than that, you should try adding an extra snack to your eating plan.)

   The basic fact of weight gain and loss is this: In order to lose weight, you must take in fewer calories than you burn. There are two ways to reach this goal. You can eat fewer calories, or you can increase the calories you burn through exercise. The Body•Mind•Life Makeover is designed to combine the two strategies—cutting your calories *and* burning off calories through exercise—with a relaxation plan to help you gain control over those weak moments when overindulgence can sabotage even your best efforts.

   Ready to get started? Before we begin, let's take a look at how the Body•Mind•Life Makeover has changed the lives of countless Slim•Fast users.

# 2

# BEFORE AND AFTER:
## SLIM•FAST
## SUCCESS STORIES

Every day, two million people in the United States use Slim•Fast products to help them lose weight, feel energized, and feel better about themselves. Over the years, the makers of Slim•Fast have received thousands of letters from consumers who have tried the plan and found that it has actually slimmed their bodies, improved their health—even changed their lives. Countless people have been motivated to begin exercising after losing weight with Slim•Fast. They've remade their eating habits, finding ways to include more fruits and vegetables into their meals and snacks. Very often they've coupled their weight-loss efforts with an exercise program that has helped them build muscle and stay fit and trim. Some letter writers have even found that Slim•Fast has given them the confidence to make major life changes— from going back to school to trying out a new career to renewing the love in their lives.

The key to success lies in making Slim•Fast part of a healthy lifestyle. In every one of these success stories, people managed to overcome the habits that kept them overweight, while incorporating new habits to keep themselves slender. What's interesting is that they all took the time to discover what worked best for them. Most remain on Slim•Fast to maintain their weight loss; others turn back to Slim•Fast to take off the 2 or 3 pounds that they gain from time to time. All of these committed dieters have resolved to live healthy by exercising, eating nutritious foods, and taking other steps to improve their lives. And, as their letters reveal, now that they've remade their bodies, they're having the time of their lives.

Another advantage of the Slim•Fast approach to weight loss is just how easy it is to use. Many dieters have found that having ready access to Slim•Fast's delicious shakes and meal bars—whether on the go or after a long day at work—makes it easier for them to stick to the plan instead of giving in to the temptations of fast or processed foods. One such success story is Marilyn Schloss from Baltimore, Maryland. In a letter to her cousin, *Makeover* coauthor Deborah Kotz, Marilyn also emphasizes the importance of exercise to the Slim•Fast Plan:

> It fits perfectly into my busy lifestyle. When I travel, I take snack and meal bars in my suitcase, so I always have something nutritious to eat on the road. At work, I pop a Slim•Fast in the freezer and eat a frozen shake with a spoon for lunch. It's very satisfying and has enabled me to lose 14 pounds, which I have been able to keep off for a year. I also find that I have more energy to exercise and have begun adding short jogging spurts to my walking routine on the treadmill. I've tried several other diet programs in the past, but I've never had as great a success maintaining my weight loss!

Sometimes losing weight can bring you closer to your loved ones and friends—especially if they act as your support system by encouraging your weight-loss efforts. You may even want to find someone to team up with. The two of you can encourage each other using the buddy system. It can also help you stay committed to your exercise plan if that someone is depending on you to show up for a workout. Bruce Mack of Clarkston, Mississippi, found that going through the Slim•Fast Makeover with his wife made losing weight fun and easy. And they got an added bonus: a stronger, happier marriage.

> I was truly on the road to self-destruction. Since our marriage in April 1994, my wife, Leslie, and I had progressively gained weight. We couldn't bear to miss our nightly dessert and sometimes an extra helping of something. As my weight soared to a personal record of 254 pounds, I could neither face my reflection in the mirror, nor tolerate the embarrass-

ment of buying size 44 jeans. Ultimately, we agreed that Slim•Fast and teamwork offered the greatest promise. Just nine months later, we're both in the best shape of our adult lives!

I went down to a size 34 pants and lost a total of 65 pounds. My wife went from a size 14 to a size 6 and lost 35 pounds. We have embraced the Slim•Fast process.

My wife and I work in the same building and spend lunch hours together whenever possible. Dashing out to a restaurant or deli, ordering, eating, and returning to the office within one hour can become a grueling task—not to mention expensive. We now enjoy a leisurely lunch of Slim•Fast at a nearby park, and we often take an invigorating walk through the park. We find that the combination of a light, nutritious meal with some exercise gives us increased energy to get through the afternoon (rather than returning from lunch weighted down like a lead balloon and ready to doze).

Once our weight decreased and our spirits increased, we began a serious exercise plan. We now have a fitness room at home with a treadmill and a variety of weights and truly cannot remember when we felt better. We also have reduced expenses dramatically—from an average of $10 per lunch every day to a mere $2. These savings offset a dinner out one night a week when we celebrate another week of success!

Most successful Slim•Fast users find that exercise speeds their weight loss and helps keep the pounds off. They also see that a combination of exercise and good eating habits gives them more energy and makes them feel healthier. Exercise, of course, also provides long-term health benefits—from reducing your risk of heart disease and diabetes to helping prevent breast, colon, and other cancers. One former exercise teacher wrote that after losing 33 pounds on Slim•Fast, she was able to jump-start her exercise regimen, and even began teaching aerobics classes again. Here's what Dinah Miller Burnette of Lewisville, North Carolina, and June Brown of Victorville, California, had to say about exercise:

I had been thin all my life—until five years ago. When my doctor prescribed a medication for an unrelated ailment, she warned me that I might gain weight as a side effect—but at that point in my life weight was the last thing I was worried about. Over the next two years I gained about 60 pounds—but it was so gradual I really didn't notice.

Then I began nursing school, where I had to sit and study—and I gained another 30 pounds. By the time I finished nursing school, I was wearing a size 24 and weighed 245 pounds. Reality hit me when my graduation pictures arrived in the mail. I couldn't believe it was really me. I woke up and said, I want my old body back.

At first, I bought the Slim•Fast powder and would make myself a shake using just the powder and skim milk, but then I learned to make wonderful shakes using the chocolate powder, a banana, skim milk, and ice, or vanilla powder, skim milk, strawberries, and ice. I drank two shakes a day, one for breakfast and one for dinner. I would eat a very low fat meal in the middle of the day, trying to have only 1,200 to 1,500 calories a day.

For exercise, I could only walk one mile a day. I was so heavy that my chest and legs ached very badly. In two months, I lost about 20 pounds, and I was very excited. When we opened our pool in the backyard, I began jogging in place in the water twenty minutes every day and continued to walk a mile and a half a day. The more I moved, the more I lost. I was learning the secret: get up, move, and eat right.

Five months after I started losing weight, I had lost almost 50 pounds, and my hairdresser (also an aerobics instructor) advised me to start light weightlifting to tone and firm my body. A fitness instructor started me on a shaping and toning regimen, and I also discovered aerobics. Now I was walking two miles a day, using Nautilus equipment every other day for about twenty minutes, and taking two to three aerobic classes each week.

A year and a half has gone by, and I can wear all my old size 9/10 clothes. I've lost 101 pounds, but I feel better than I used to be at this size because I'm exercising and eating right. I have discovered that it's not enough to be thin—you have to be active at whatever size you are.

I have so much energy now, I feel like a nineteen-year-old. I plan to make eating right and exercise a permanent part of my lifestyle. I use the canned ready-to-drink Slim•Fast shakes; they're so convenient to throw in my lunch bag with a banana and apple. I now walk three miles every day and continue to lift weights. Persistence really pays off. I am walking proof of that.

My name is June Brown, and I lost 100 pounds thanks to Slim•Fast!

I'd been afraid to step on the scale for so many years. After high school my weight had slowly begun to climb. But I'm five feet nine inches and big boned, and people always told me I could carry the weight. Being a seamstress also helped me to overlook my true size; I was always able to make my clothes bigger. Over the years, I tried and tried again to diet down to an acceptable weight, only to have it come right back. Then, in 1987, I got pregnant after trying unsuccessfully for three years. The weight from my second pregnancy didn't come off easily; it climbed from 185 to my heaviest, 245 pounds.

Two and a half years ago, I was a size 24. For Christmas that year, I bought myself a treadmill and began what would end up as my new lifestyle. When I first stepped on it, I stumbled several times and was only able to stay on for two to three minutes. The next day, I tried again and stayed on without falling. Keeping at it the next few days brought increased self-esteem. I was able to walk for up to ten minutes.

Since I was doing so well with the exercise, I thought I would cut my food intake and look at my eating habits (which weren't very good). I began to drink Slim•Fast in the morning and at lunch. It was so easy, and the snack bars were very tasty whenever I needed a snack. I soon found that if I cut out the fats, reduced the calories, and increased exercise, I would lose weight. I then started to enhance my old recipes to be fat free (or close to it). I used to cook with a lot of oil, but I learned to substitute cooking spray when frying and applesauce when baking. After two months, I added a variety of breakfast and lunch menus and began to do more exercise. My kids even started doing exercise videos with me.

Within three months of adopting my new lifestyle, I stepped on the scale and was surprised to find it went only to 209. I was elated. My husband and people at work began to see a difference. My eleventh anniversary was approaching, and I was determined to fit into my size 14 wedding dress. I increased my exercise to a daily half-hour walk at work and an aerobic video three to four nights a week.

On April 28, when my anniversary arrived, I had the perfect evening planned. With candlelight and a romantic dinner ready, my husband was shocked to see me in my wedding dress (which now fit—a little snug, but I was able to zip it up).

By the end of July 1995 I'd reached my original goal of 160 pounds and a dress size of 10. Since then, I've lost another 15 pounds and can fit into a size 8. Coworkers, friends, and relatives are always asking for my recipes. They all want to know what diet I found. I tell them it's not a diet, it's a new lifestyle. A year and a half later, I'm still at my goal. I have so much more energy. There is nothing I can't do.

Sometimes gaining weight and feeling bad about yourself can become a vicious cycle; you overeat, you put on pounds, you dislike the way you look, then you eat more to make yourself feel better. But Slim•Fast can help you break that cycle forever, as Sheila Silver of Norfolk, Virginia, reports:

I am a twenty-four-year-old nurse who managed to go from 95 pounds on her wedding day to 274 pounds five years later. Now, even though I gave birth to four beautiful children in that time frame, I must admit that they weren't to blame for my enormous weight gain. An insatiable appetite, and no control over my eating habits, were the culprits. Having a family history of high blood pressure and stroke, I had tried plenty of fad diets, pills, and creams; I'd even thought seriously about a gastric bypass! You name it, I'd probably tried it.

Then one day last August, while sitting on my bed finishing off a bag of chips and Pecan Sandies (my daily routine), a television commercial for Slim•Fast caught my eye. The woman told of how she'd lost 20 pounds in just six short months on the Slim•Fast Plan. For a split second I felt a glimmer of hope; but then I began to rationalize, thinking that even if it did work it was probably only good for people like her who needed to lose only 20 or 30 pounds—not for me, who needed to lose 100 pounds or more. So I got up to go to the kitchen to grab another bag of chips. And in doing so I caught a glimpse of myself in my full-length bedroom mirror. I looked like a female sumo wrestler! I stared in disbelief. How could I have let this happen?

That next morning I had my first frozen strawberry Slim•Fast shake, while reading the meal suggestions in the brochure enclosed in the can of powdered Slim•Fast. A shake for breakfast, a shake for lunch, and a sensible dinner of my choice—I could do this!

And by the end of that first month I had lost over 10 pounds! But I knew I still had a long, long way to go, so I continued to have my morning and noon shakes, followed by a balanced meal in the evenings—not forgetting to include six to eight glasses of water daily. Six months later I had lost over 50 pounds on the Slim•Fast Plan! And I honestly didn't even miss my food binges, because I never felt depressed or hungry.

I've continued to lose a steady 2 to 3 pounds a week, dropping from a size 22 to size 14 and then, finally, to size 5! Just this morning I took a trip to the department store to buy a dress, and returned to the register with two of the most darling outfits you've ever seen. The store clerk looked at the clothes and then looked at me; finally, she said, "Honey, these are going to be a mite big on you. Why don't you go back and get a smaller size?"

I weigh 125 pounds now—more than 140 pounds less than I weighed when I began. I want everyone to know that you don't have to be a celebrity or have a personal trainer or spend your money on expensive diet programs that don't even work. All you need is a sensible plan.

For many dieters, the energy gain they get through the Slim•Fast lifestyle is just as important as the cosmetic benefits of weight loss. Take Pam Andrews of Gordon, Alabama:

> I am fifty-three years old and had a weight problem my whole life. I've tried numerous diets and rode the "lose-and-gain cycle" until I was dizzy! Then about five years ago I gave Slim•Fast a try, hoping to lose at least 19 pounds by the time Christmas came around. I didn't want to attend another festive party in the predictable tent fashions I had worn in the past. Following the Slim•Fast program, I reached my goal and didn't have to go hungry or feel deprived to do it. I went on to lose the rest of the weight I needed to take off—another 31 pounds—and have maintained my weight just by supplementing with Slim•Fast from time to time.
>
> I have an animal shelter with about two hundred dogs and some cats; sometimes we even take in rabbits, turtles, and birds. Most of them come from the highways and byways, where they were abandoned or lost their way. We take care of them, give them love, and restore them to health. We try to find new homes for them, but many become permanent residents of our country home. I also work with elderly people, homeless people, and people coping with substance-abuse problems. As you can see, my day requires a lot of energy, which most dieting regimens can sap. When I need to cut calories, Slim•Fast lets me do it without sacrificing energy. I'm a good example that you can be fit, trim, and even sexy well past forty!

Losing excess pounds is one of the single best things you can do for your health. Even a modest weight loss of 5 to 10 percent of your body weight can improve your health by leaps and bounds. Examples of ways to improve your health by losing weight include lowering the risk of heart disease by improving blood pressure and cholesterol levels; reducing chances of developing diabetes; and eliminating the bodily aches and pains that come with being overweight. Even if you have no medical problems, you'll be amazed at how much better you feel after you achieve a healthier weight—like Jon Kouba of Rapid City, South Dakota:

I'm a single, twenty-four-year-old male college student who has been working three jobs to put myself through school. As a morbidly obese person, 285 pounds overweight, I kept a painstaking, extremely accurate daily journal of everything that happened in my efforts to lose weight—efforts that included the Slim•Fast program.

I kept track of the exact foods I ate, the exact calories and fat grams; I kept track of my daily weight and the lost inches on different parts of my body; I kept track of my emotions, battles, successes, and exact details of my exercise regimen. I was so determined from day one that I lose this weight that it showed in my dedication in keeping my records from the very first day onward. I still have the first Slim•Fast shake can's lid tab that I hung on my wall to keep me focused.

Obviously, there was a lot more to my diet than just Slim•Fast—like hard work, patience, dedication, perseverance, and hard exercise. I also changed to healthy eating patterns that included lots of fruits and vegetables. But I still owe a big debt of gratitude to your wonderful product. Most people would say that I am attractive, happy, and filled with tons of energy—unlike the person I was at my very worst. I have an incredibly strong heart rate and extremely low cholesterol and am probably in the best shape of my life. I truly, truly love your product.

For some people, the Slim•Fast Makeover has even opened the door to a new career, giving them the confidence and motivation they needed to launch themselves into a new stage of life. Linda Adams is one of those.

After my husband passed away two years ago it was necessary that I go back to work. They weren't exactly beating down the door to hire a sixty-year-old woman back into the hotel business. For professional reasons and to regain my self-esteem, I embarked on a self-improvement program. When I'm at home, I prepare my Slim•Fast and a banana each morning for breakfast. On the road I freeze a can of Slim•Fast, and by the time it thaws out I'm ready for my lunch drink.

In a year and a half, I've gone from 196 to 139 pounds, returned to work as director of sales and marketing in a hotel, and have again assembled a career wardrobe. I love salads and usually get hungry around 2:00 P.M., so I indulge in my favorite chicken Caesar salad. I eat what I want, but only half as much as I used to. I also keep an eye on fat content.

I walk and ride my bike nearly every day for two miles. I feel great, and my five grandkids think I'm thirty-seven. My friends are in absolute awe of the transformation.

And, finally, here's an extraordinary story that proves it's never too late to start changing your life:

Gentlemen:

I was born in 1910. On September 7, 1999, I will be eighty-nine, but that sounds so hollow to me now: I am not as old now, at eighty-nine, as I was at seventy-five.

In the course of my life as a businessman, I found that the pressures and demands of my career just gave me no time to think of caring for my own body. Year after year there were business dinners and lunches that sometimes included a cocktail, and in the evening I would go home to a wonderful wife who was a good cook and thought it was her lot at least to provide me with lots of good food.

Yes, it happened—I gained weight, to the shameful total of 242 pounds. One morning, as I was dressing, I happened to stray over in front of the large mirror; I couldn't help but look—but I was appalled at what I saw. I called in to the office and told them I wouldn't be coming in that day. I went to the neighborhood grocery and purchased a few cans of Slim•Fast. Then I made a chart covering fifty-two weeks; at the top left was my present weight and at the lower right was my goal, which was 165.

Slim•Fast and I went to work, and how beautifully satisfying it was to weigh in every morning and see my weight go down! I did a modest exercise practice that I continue even today; I walked or jogged from four to six miles a day; and by the end of the year I had lost the weight I'd promised myself—with hardly any loose skin to worry about. My belts have an extra twelve inches, but I still use them all—they remind me every day of what I've accomplished.

My wife passed away two years ago, but I'm enclosing a photo of my new lady friend. I do believe I've turned the clock back many years by using Slim•Fast, and she's as grateful as I am about the results. Thank you for giving me "another life"—one perhaps shorter than the first, but just as precious.

Sincerely,
William Dale Opperman, Yankton, South Dakota

# Success Story in the Town of Pound

In 1992, the tiny town of Pound, Wisconsin, decided to accept an exciting challenge from the Slim•Fast Foods Company. Slim•Fast offered to provide free shakes and snack bars to anyone in the town who was interested in losing weight. More than a quarter of the town's adult population—158 people—decided to enroll in the study to see how much weight they could lose. They were allowed to have two Ultra Slim•Fast shakes a day, plus a well-balanced low-fat meal for dinner and up to three Ultra Slim•Fast snacks or fruit. They were also encouraged to exercise.

After four months, tabloid headlines blared "Town Loses a Ton and a Half!" The residents, almost all of whom remained with the program, lost a whopping 2,869 pounds—an average loss of 18 pounds a person. Then-mayor Richard Adamski, who lost 42 pounds himself, declared, "At this rate, the town of Pound will soon be Ounces!"

Five years later, more than 92 percent of the original participants were still using Slim•Fast; women had kept off an average of 9 pounds, men an average of 13. What's more, 80 percent of the participants stayed well below their starting weight after five years. Meanwhile, a control group of participants from the nearby areas who did not take Slim•Fast *gained* an average of 14 pounds during these five years. These results were collected as part of an ongoing research study and were recently published in the prestigious scientific journal *Nutrition*.

Karen Supita, who participated in the study, recently wrote Slim•Fast to thank them for the success she's had as a result of starting the plan. "Little did I realize when I started on the Slim•Fast program over seven and a half years ago that my entire life and lifestyle would be changed from then on. I'd gone from a size 8 to a size 16 in less than a year. Then I started on the program, and made Slim•Fast and exercise a routine part of my day. As I stuck to the diet and the weight began to come off, my energy level rose in direct proportion. It wasn't long before I'd slimmed down and shaped up and returned to a size 8! Slim•Fast has changed my life and, I very happily say, for the better."

Another participant found that she was able to actually leave her house again after losing some excess weight. "When the diet started, I weighed in at 313 pounds," said Virginia Miller, a fifty-eight-year-old grandmother. "I'm five feet four inches, and I felt like a blimp. I was so embarrassed by my size. I hated to go outside because I thought everyone was laughing at me. Now I walk three miles every night. I even go to the community center and work out on one of the four treadmills Slim•Fast donated to Pound. I feel like a whole new person. It's wonderful."

Dana Rothacker, Ph.D., who continues to conduct the study in Pound, visits Pound every six months to conduct weigh-ins and monitor the town's weight-loss and weight-maintenance efforts. "We don't provide counseling or nutritional advice—aside from the instructions on the package," she said. "We wanted to see how Slim•Fast is used in the real world, and we see that it works!"

# Five Habits of Successful Dieters

Research suggests that the vast majority of people who lose weight through a weight-loss program wind up gaining back the weight within three to five years. Rather than trying to figure out what the majority are doing wrong, a group of researchers decided to determine what the most successful dieters are doing right. According to a study conducted by the University of Pittsburgh Medical Center and the University of Colorado Health Sciences Center, those dieters who are best able to keep the weight off tend to have modified their behavior as well as simply changing their eating habits—that is, they change their bodies by changing their lives. A significant portion of people in the study used meal replacements like Slim•Fast to help lose weight and maintain the loss; the average dieter lost an average of 37 pounds and maintained it over seven years. Here are a few specific strategies successful weight maintainers in the study used:

**Restricting fat intake:** Successful dieters avoided fried foods and substituted low-fat for high-fat products. "It is likely that the majority of maintainers obtain less than 30% of calories from fat," conclude the study authors.

**Engaging in strenuous exercise:** Although everyone in the study did some form of mild or moderate activity, the successful weight maintainers engaged in more strenuous activities (running, weightlifting, aerobics) and more activities that made them sweat. Fifty-two percent of the maintainers reported working out strenuously three or more times a week.

**Frequent weigh-ins:** About 55 percent of the successful weight maintainers weighed themselves at least once a week. In another study, researchers found that 75 percent of successful dieters weighed themselves at least once a week. This kind of regular monitoring is clearly necessary for those who want to control their weight.

**Less TV:** The weight maintainers watched an average of 13.7 hours of TV each week. Regainers, on the other hand, watched an average of 15.2 hours. Perhaps the maintainers spent the extra ninety minutes sweating through their workouts, rather than sitting on the couch.

**Seeking out a prescribed method or weight-loss program:** Just 26 percent of weight-loss maintainers lost weight on their own. The rest used a diet or medicine prescribed by their physician, a commercial program, or meal replacements such as Slim•Fast.

Now that you know the basics of the Slim•Fast Makeover and you've seen how it has helped countless dieters achieve the body, mind, and life they want, it's time to make a decision. Are you ready to give yourself a makeover? Only you can decide when you're ready to make a change, but getting started sooner is almost always easier than putting things off until "just the right moment."

Put a little trust in yourself. You won't let yourself down.

# 3

## 14 DAYS
## TO A NEW YOU!

When NASA's engineers designed the *Apollo 11* spacecraft, they had one central challenge: They had to launch the craft with enough speed and power so that it would not only lift off the ground, but break free from the Earth's gravitational pull. It took an enormous hydrogen reaction to propel the rocket around the Earth and out of its orbit, sending the rocket aloft and into the heavens.

Well, if you can think of your body as the rocket, the Slim•Fast 14-Day Plan is the fuel that will blast you off to weight loss and good health. The initial momentum you'll build on the 14-Day Plan will give you the speed you need to help you reach your ultimate goal: a healthy weight and a healthy body. Once you get that momentum going, you'll see how easy it is to change your life forever.

The point of the 14-Day Plan is to show you how great you can feel once you start eating nutritious foods, exercising, and managing the stress in your life. Each of these three components works together to maximize your weight-loss efforts, while improving your health at the same time. Do you sometimes get moody or irritable for no real reason? You'll feel better as you fuel your body with high-quality foods and exercise. Prone to afternoon slumps? You'll feel more energy throughout the day—and even the fact that you're taking your health in your own hands should invigorate your spirits.

# How Much Weight Will You Lose?

Although weight loss varies from person to person, you can lose up to 3 to 4 pounds while you're on the 14-Day Plan. Assuming that you normally eat around 2,500 calories a day, the plan trims off 1,000 to 1,100 calories, getting you down to a reasonable intake of 1,400 to 1,500. And here's the simple-math way it works: Since the average dieter loses a pound of fat for every 3,500 calories burned, reducing your intake by 1,000 calories a day will enable you to shed 1 pound every three or four days. And on top of that basic weight loss, most people lose about a pound or two of water when they first begin a weight-loss plan: the large amounts of bread, pasta, and other starchy carbohydrates we typically eat cause the body to retain excess water, and cutting down on the starches should help you lose a measurable amount of water weight.

Losing 4 pounds in just two weeks can give you the motivation you'll need to continue the healthy habits you began on the 14-Day Plan. And if there's anything that's important in losing weight, it's motivation. That's why the 14-Day Plan is so useful. It can help you start replacing your old habits with a new healthy lifestyle—*without any major planning on your part*. All you have to do is take a ready-made shopping list to the supermarket, slip into some comfortable exercise clothes for a moderate workout, and follow a lifestyle plan that's enjoyable and rewarding. Soon you'll see that losing weight is more than a dream—it's absolutely within your grasp. Just get your body moving, take some relaxation time for yourself, and follow the simple Slim•Fast eating plan.

# Sound Science, No Gimmicks

Sure, the 14-Day Plan sounds great. But how does it work?

The answer is simple: Each of the plan's elements is based on sound science. *Slim•Fast meal replacements*—Slim•Fast and Ultra Slim•Fast shakes and Meal On-The-Go Bars—replace the high-calorie meals we're all used to eating with a great-tasting, satisfying alternative. When combined with a sensible meal and snacks, they provide the balanced nutrition you need to feel satisfied and energized on fewer calories. And they contain no appetite suppressants, fat-burning chemicals, or drugs of any kind. The *exercise must-dos* give you a selection of strategies to help boost your body's metabolism, so you'll burn more calories and lose weight faster. And the *instant stress relievers* will give you a mini-vacation every day from life's little aggravations—the daily distractions that can sabotage your weight-loss efforts by undermining your motivation and sending you back to the freezer for another tasty helping of high-calorie comfort food.

The proper balance of nutrition, exercise, and relaxation you'll get on the 14-Day Plan will help you balance your body's systems. Your digestive system can run more smoothly, since you'll be eating smaller meals more frequently throughout the day; you'll be less likely to experience heartburn and other symptoms of indigestion, and the added fiber in the Slim•Fast Plan will help prevent constipation. You can also experience more energy as your body becomes better at absorbing the balanced level of nutrients in your diet—and as your circulation improves through exercise and relaxation.

In short, your body will finally be working *for* you instead of against you—retraining itself, through your new lifestyle, to help you live the life you want.

## Quitting Smoking—*My* First Lesson in Getting Healthy

In the fall of 1997, having quit for a decade, I found myself smoking again. It was a weak-willed response to the stress of having two TV series at once, and I knew I couldn't let it last very long. (This was especially true because cigarettes shouldn't be combined with the estrogen included in hormone-replacement therapy, which I take religiously.)

But I already weighed close to 140 pounds, and I was afraid that quitting would push my weight even higher. I was playing a mental shell-game on myself, using my concerns about weight gain to keep smoking—telling myself I'd be eating my way out of a career if I didn't. In my heart of hearts, though, I knew better.

So when I saw an ad for the Duke Diet and Fitness Center and found out they could help people quit smoking *and* take off weight, I couldn't resist. (For one thing, the irony was too great—Duke is located right in Durham, North Carolina, the heart of tobacco country.) I spent three weeks there, quit smoking for good, even lost a few pounds—and had one of the most interesting times of my life.

The dining facilities at Duke are all communal; you eat all your meals together at group tables, with people of all ages (from eighteen to seventy!) and backgrounds all wearing jogging shorts or exercise suits, eating together as if they'd all been thrown together into one big all-inclusive school cafeteria. Since I was cold-turkeying off cigarettes, I told myself, the last thing I wanted to do was make new friends; I figured I'd just hunker down, keep to myself, and get out, and for the first few days I did.

But then, on the morning of my fourth smoke-free day, I was bounding up the front steps when I was confronted by the wide grin of Maurice, a big twenty-year-old kid from San Francisco. Parked in front of the entrance like a temple guardian, he said, "Morning, Lauren. Sleep well? Here, let me introduce you to some of my friends." And with that my shyness chains broke. Maurice must have been over 300 pounds; he and Abner, a 400-pound-plus ex-chef, were my first buddies there. They were such kind, open guys that they made me stop and think about the real reasons I hadn't been talking to anyone the first few days. And the answer came back: People with severe weight problems, I found, struck fear into my heart. They were like pain made manifest; I felt as if their bodies were carrying the suffering of their souls. I couldn't face pain that obvious, because I knew I had similar pain myself, and I'd always dealt with that pain by hiding it, silently and invisibly, on my own.

Once I faced down my prejudices—thanks to Maurice and his pals—my life at the center changed. I got into everyone's business, and they got into mine. Sometimes it felt like we were a combat team fighting for survival together.

After a while, I decided that one thing I could contribute would be to offer a series of makeup-application classes. I figured that in a place where so many women were managing to lose weight—from 8 pounds to 50—there'd be plenty of interest in a quick class that could teach them how to make their new selves look as glamorous as possible. What were scheduled as hour-long classes ended up running for three; they became half instruction and half stand-up routine, as I kept joking and working till everyone had a chance. And the letters of appreciation I got afterward were wonderful.

After three weeks at Duke, I emerged a happy and smoke-free camper. But the most important thing I took away from my time there was that changing your lifestyle—whether it's quitting smoking, losing weight, or anything else—is a job you can *only* do yourself. The center offers one intensive way to do it, in which you take time off and devote all your energies to one goal. The Slim•Fast Makeover helps you achieve the same goal by making just a few changes within your everyday life. All it takes is the desire to change.

# 14 Days of Eating Right

The Slim•Fast Plan, with its basic 1,400- to 1,500-calorie daily allowance, is simple and easy to follow. It also gives you the most nutritious foods for the fewest amount of calories. Unlike many other calorie-restricted diets, which require you to guesstimate the number of calories you're consuming, the Slim•Fast Plan takes away the guesswork and enables you to eat the actual number of calories on the plan.

At the center of the plan is the balanced, medically proven combination of vitamins, minerals, and other nutrients that goes into every Slim•Fast product. Each day on the plan you'll be drinking two great-tasting Slim•Fast shakes (or eating two Meal On-The-Go Bars) a day plus a Slim•Fast snack bar between meals. One shake provides one-third of your daily requirements for most vitamins and minerals. It also provides the right amounts of fiber, protein, and carbohydrates, along with a small amount of fat, for a total of 200 to 220 calories. The meal-replacement system gives you a way to get the nutrients you need, with a limited number of calories, without depriving you of the pleasures of eating. And the proper balance of nutrients in Slim•Fast products will help your body absorb nutrients more efficiently.

But don't worry—there's more to the eating plan than just shakes and bars. The 14-Day Plan includes a sensible dinner every night, and provides for snacking throughout the day—a program based on sensible dietary guidelines established by the U.S. Department of Agriculture. These guidelines call for eating a variety of foods in order to get the forty nutrients (such as vitamins, minerals, protein, and fiber) that are essential for good health. And they emphasize that no single food can provide all the nutrients in the amounts you need. They recommend that 30 percent or less of your total daily calories come from fat, that 20 percent of your calories come from protein, and that 50 percent come from carbohydrates (fruits, vegetables, milk sugars, sweeteners, and starches).

To help you meet those guidelines every day, each day of the 14-Day Plan includes a series of recipes and snacking suggestions—featuring several servings of vegetables as well as a fiber-rich starch. The recipes also contain ample amounts of heart-healthy proteins such as fish, white-meat poultry, lean cuts of meat, and beans. Oils and other fats are used sparingly, and fresh fruit is featured for dessert.

Combine these dinners with two Slim•Fast meal-replacement shakes or bars, three fresh fruit snacks, and a Slim•Fast snack bar, and your total calorie intake for the day will be around 1,400 to 1,500 calories. This is a perfect eating plan for losing weight slowly and steadily—on the order of 1 to 2 pounds a week. That's the safest and most effective way to lose weight, according to health experts.

The 14-Day Plan also emphasizes another major nutrient: fiber. Fiber helps combat such health ills as colorectal cancer, gastrointestinal disorders, diabetes, and heart disease—and, because it makes you feel full more quickly, fiber can also help you curb overeating. Each Slim•Fast shake contains up to 5 grams of fiber; two shakes plus the fruits, vegetables, and grains recommended on the plan will make it easy to meet the daily intake of 20 to 35 grams recommended by the American Dietetic Association and the National Cancer Institute.

In simple terms, the 14-Day Plan will very likely have you eating better than you have in years. After all, most of us eat fewer than five servings of fruits and vegetables a day. And the average American ingests only 5 to 13 grams of fiber a day—less than a third of the recommended amount. When you consider that you're probably not getting enough calcium and other essential vitamins and minerals—or enough phytochemicals, the disease-fighting nutrients found in fruits and vegetables—you'll realize how much you have to gain from trying the plan.

The 14-Day Plan will also teach you cooking tricks to help you save on fat and calories. The recipes all emphasize healthy cooking techniques: Foods are grilled, steamed, broiled, and baked—not fried. Nonstick low-calorie cooking sprays are used to coat pans instead of oil. Dressings for salads are fat-free or reduced-calorie. The protein choices include lean cuts of meat, white-meat chicken and turkey, and fish, to help you get the greatest helpings of nutrients with the least amount of saturated fat. Vegetables are a prominent part of every meal, and fruit plays a starring role at dessert.

Here's a quick rundown of the plan you'll be following. It's been tested by millions of Slim•Fast users, and it works!

To help you lose weight, the plan calls for you to replace two regular meals a day with Slim•Fast shakes or meal bars; to snack lightly throughout the day on fruit, vegetables, or Slim•Fast snack bars; and to finish it all off with a sensible dinner. Here's the basic Weight-Loss Plan:

*To lose weight, just remember:*

### Shake • Shake • Meal

**BREAKFAST:** 1 Slim•Fast Shake or Meal On-The-Go Bar

**SNACK:** 1 piece of fruit *or* 1 cup raw vegetables

**LUNCH:** 1 Slim•Fast Shake or Meal On-The-Go Bar

**SNACK:** 1 piece of fruit *or* 1 cup raw vegetables

**SNACK:** 1 Slim•Fast Nutritional Energy Bar *or* 1 serving nonfat yogurt

**DINNER:** 1 large tossed salad; 6 ounces of protein (meat, chicken, fish, or soy/vegetable protein); 3 servings of cooked or steamed vegetables; 1 serving of starch ($1/2$ baked potato, 1 small ear of corn, or $1/2$ cup rice or pasta); 1 piece of fruit for dessert

*Important:* On the Slim•Fast Plan, it's crucial to drink eight glasses of water (or another caffeine-free, noncaloric beverage) each day to keep your body hydrated. You can still drink caffeinated coffee, tea, or diet colas, but don't count them toward your water amount because the caffeine they contain tends to dehydrate the body.

Once you've finished losing the weight you want—whether it's 4 pounds you lost on the 14-Day Plan or another 20 you lost by staying on the plan until you reached your goal—it's important to keep up your efforts. The Slim•Fast Plan makes it easy to keep your weight in check with the Weight Maintenance Plan, which calls for two sensible meals and one shake or meal bar per day.

*To maintain your ideal weight, remember:*

## Meal • Shake • Meal

**BREAKFAST:** 1 bowl (1 ounce) high-fiber cereal; 1/2 cup fat-free milk; 1/2 cup nonfat yogurt; 1 piece fruit; *or* 1 Slim•Fast Shake or Meal On-The-Go Bar

**SNACK:** 1 piece of fruit

**LUNCH:** 2 ounces luncheon meat or cheese; 3 servings vegetables (lettuce, shredded carrots, tomato slices, etc.); 2 slices whole-wheat bread; 1 cup nonfat yogurt, 1/2 melon, or fruit cup; *or* 1 Slim•Fast Shake or Meal On-The-Go Bar

**SNACK:** 1 piece of fruit

**SNACK:** 1 Slim•Fast Nutritional Energy Bar *or* 1 serving nonfat yogurt

**DINNER:** Vegetable soup or side salad; 6 ounces of protein (meat, chicken, fish, or soy/vegetable protein); 3 servings of cooked or steamed vegetables; 1 serving of starch (potato, rice, pasta, etc.); 1 piece of fruit for dessert

The chapter that follows includes quick and delicious recipes for each day of the 14-Day Plan to help you make your weight-loss efforts as easy and satisfying as possible.

# Fit, Fabulous, and Fun

Along with mouth-watering menus, each day of the 14-Day Plan includes what we call an *exercise must-do*. These exercises are designed to give you a mixture of cardiovascular activity (steady exercise that works your heart muscle and makes you sweat), resistance training (toning exercises to strengthen your muscles), and stretching techniques (exercises that increase flexibility and balance). The exercises change every day, so you won't get bored doing the same thing over and over; there's something to fit everyone's tastes to help you find the exercises you enjoy most—and thus will be most likely to come back to on a permanent basis.

The goal of the exercise portion of the plan is to get your body moving for an hour every day. That might sound like a lot at first—but if you break it up into manageable mini-workouts throughout the day, you can accomplish a lot even if you can't steal a full hour away. And it's even easier if you can find ways to walk or bike instead of driving during the course of your regular day. So supplement the exercise tips on the 14-Day Plan with a little moving of your own. Whether it's bopping around the house to your favorite CD or playing a game of tag with your kids, you should be having fun and getting active at the same time.

You might ask: Do I really need to exercise if I can lose weight on the Slim•Fast Plan alone? For your answer, consider some of the health benefits of exercise:

**Increases metabolic rate.** It's one of the paradoxes of dieting: The less you eat and the less you weigh, the lower your metabolism—the rate at which your body burns calories. Thus, you need to eat less to maintain your loss, and even less to keep losing weight. Exercise helps counteract this problem by speeding up your metabolism—during your workouts and for several hours afterward.

**Counteracts the health ills of obesity.** Exercise can help alleviate many of the health problems that come with being overweight. It can reduce your risk of heart disease by improving blood pressure and cholesterol levels. It can help stabilize blood sugar and reduce insulin resistance, to lower your risk of diabetes. It gives you energy by improving the circulation of your blood. And by strengthening your muscles, it helps alleviate joint problems that result from carrying too much excess weight.

**Helps control appetite.** Studies with both animals and humans suggest that exercise can help control appetite—at least when you work out moderately. Unfortunately, many of us tend to reward ourselves after a workout with "just a taste" of the wrong kind of food—and it takes only a few cookies to add back the calories you just burned. Beware the urge to splurge—that's your mind talking, not your body.

**Preserves the body's muscle.** The fact is, your body tends to lose muscle as well as fat when you lose weight. Exercise can help maximize fat loss while limiting muscle loss; combining exercise with diet does this more effectively than diet alone.

**Improves confidence and psychological factors.** There's no quicker route to a better body image—and greater confidence—than exercise. Just the fact that you're making positive changes can boost your spirits, and as you see your body becoming more toned and fit your self-confidence is sure to follow. Research also suggests that exercise helps at the hormonal level, increasing your "feel-good" endorphins and reducing stress hormones. Exercise can also be a great stress reliever if you're used to eating when you're tense—and that can only bolster your weight-loss efforts.

**Increases your chances of long-term success.** As we've seen, studies show that exercise is the most important factor in determining how well dieters maintain weight loss. It's simple: stay with the exercise program, and you'll help those pounds stay off.

# Nurture Yourself

The third element of the 14-Day Plan is the *instant stress reliever* included for each day of the plan. The truth is, the only smart way to remake your body and life is to pay equal attention to remaking your mind—taking the time to care for the inner you. It might surprise you that a weight-loss plan would devote much time to something as natural as relaxation; after all, most of us lead such busy lives that we'd never dream we'd need help to learn to relax. After all, you might think, who needs lessons in relaxation if I already spend an hour or two every night vegging out in front of the TV?

Once you've tried the relaxation techniques on the 14-Day Plan, though, you'll realize the difference between being a couch potato and practicing high-quality relaxation. The best relaxation leaves you feeling refreshed because you've taken the time to focus on clearing your head of your daily stresses, and releasing the tensions that you've built up over the course of a stressful day. Instead of settling for sneaking half an hour of rest in between tense moments—distracting yourself for half an hour with a magazine, say, before getting up to make dinner—on the 14-Day Plan you'll learn to free yourself from your daily tensions and renew your spirit.

Not convinced? Consider the multitude of research findings on how stress affects your weight and the onset of weight-related illnesses.

- Previous dieters who described themselves as stressed are much more likely to regain the weight they've lost than those who aren't as stressed, according to researchers from the Miriam Hospital in Rhode Island.
- Healthy people who say they frequently express anger or hostility have significantly higher blood sugar than more relaxed dieters, according to a study from the University of Washington, Seattle. This makes them more prone to eating binges—and puts them at higher risk for diabetes.
- In a study of five hundred normal-weight and overweight adults, researchers from the Baylor College of Medicine in Houston, Texas, found that those who were most likely to maintain stable weights had a greater general sense of well-being and lower stress levels than those whose weight yo-yoed up and down the scale.

Now you're ready to begin the 14-Day Plan. It's time to make some sensible changes to your way of living, to improve your health and create a happier life for yourself. It's time to give yourself a makeover—inside and out, body, mind, and life.

So what are you waiting for?

# The Importance of Sleep

Too many of us assume we can get by with as little as five or six hours of sleep a night—going to bed at 12:30 A.M., say, and getting up at 6:30. But the truth is, very few people can function well on that little sleep. Most adults need seven to nine hours a night to achieve optimal rest. Researchers believe that sleep is our body's most important period of rest and recovery, restoring the brain and body after the normal stresses of daily activity. Getting too little sleep can impair your ability to concentrate, cause memory problems, and make you feel drowsy and moody throughout the day. Some studies even suggest that getting too little sleep can shorten your life span.

Getting the right amount of sleep is essential during the 14-Day Plan. Even if you're following the plan to the letter, you won't get the energy boost you should, or feel as great as you can, if you aren't getting enough sleep. What's more, sleep scientists now know it's not enough just to lie in bed and rest; to get the most out of our slumber, we need *quality* sleep as well as quantity. Here's how to get the kind of sleep you need:

**Keep your room cool.** Studies are clear that sleep is improved if the room temperature is on the low side—from 60 to 65 degrees Fahrenheit.

**Use your bed only for sleeping (and lovemaking).** Balancing your checkbook or doing work in bed brings stress in where it doesn't belong. Do your work in another room—and well before bedtime, so you'll be fully relaxed when you hit the pillow.

**Take a short nap (if you need one) early in the day.** Never nap after 2:00 P.M. or for longer than an hour. Taking longer, later naps can leave you less tired at night, hampering your ability to get a deep, full night's sleep.

**Avoid alcohol within two hours of bedtime.** Although it's a depressant, alcohol interferes with sleep by disrupting your sleep patterns, particularly in the second half of the night. Drinking may help you fall asleep more easily, but you won't sleep as deeply or soundly.

**Keep a regular sleep schedule.** Go to sleep and wake up around the same time each day. Going to bed late and sleeping in two days in a row (over the weekend, for

**Before**

# Slim·Fast®
## *Success Stories*

**After**

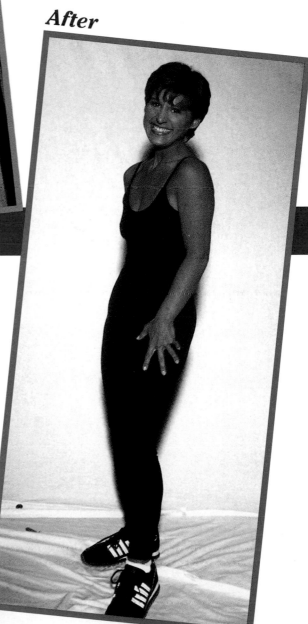

**G**ina Spillari-Melendez of Little Rock, Arkansas, had been heavy all her life, and was never very happy; she always felt as though she were living "in a shell" that prevented her from leading a fun and active life. When she lost over 50 pounds in six months, her whole attitude changed; she was able to start doing all the things she'd always wanted to do. Gina has kept her weight off for six years now, and she vows that she'll never be heavy again.

Results not typical.

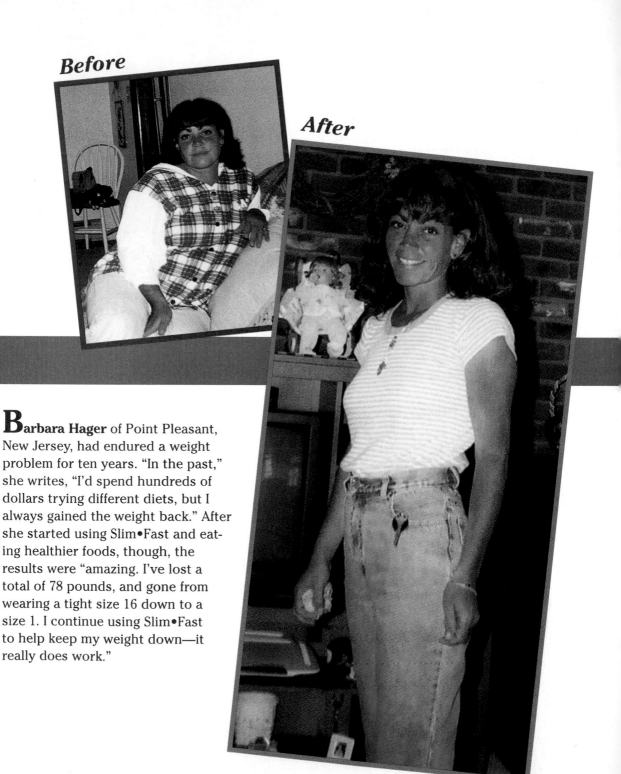

*Before*

*After*

**B**arbara **Hager** of Point Pleasant, New Jersey, had endured a weight problem for ten years. "In the past," she writes, "I'd spend hundreds of dollars trying different diets, but I always gained the weight back." After she started using Slim•Fast and eating healthier foods, though, the results were "amazing. I've lost a total of 78 pounds, and gone from wearing a tight size 16 down to a size 1. I continue using Slim•Fast to help keep my weight down—it really does work."

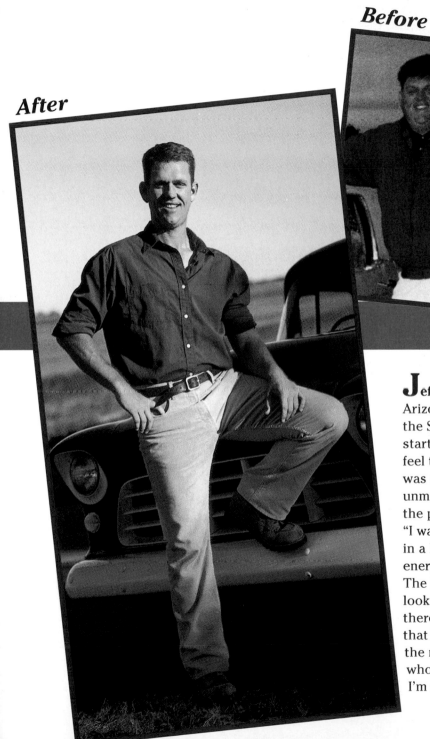

**After**

**Before**

**J**eff Showalter of Tucson, Arizona, lost over 100 pounds on the Slim•Fast Plan. "Before I started the plan, I really didn't feel there was much to live for. I was really overweight, unhealthy, unmotivated." After he started the plan, everything changed. "I was able to drop the weight in a healthy way, increase my energy levels, and change my life. The best part for me is that I look great, I feel great, and there's nothing in this world that I can't do. When I look in the mirror, I see somebody who's got a lot of confidence. I'm ecstatic."

**Before**

**After**

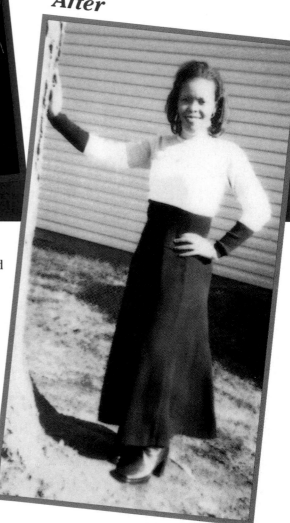

**S**heila Silver of Norfolk, Virginia, has managed to lose 140 pounds using the Slim•Fast Plan. "I don't even look like the same miserable person I was," she writes. "And if it weren't for the photos, I probably wouldn't even have believed I was that big. I want everyone to see and hear about my success with the Slim•Fast Plan, so they'll know that you don't have to be a celebrity or have a personal trainer or spend your money on expensive diet programs, when you can do it with just two shakes a day."

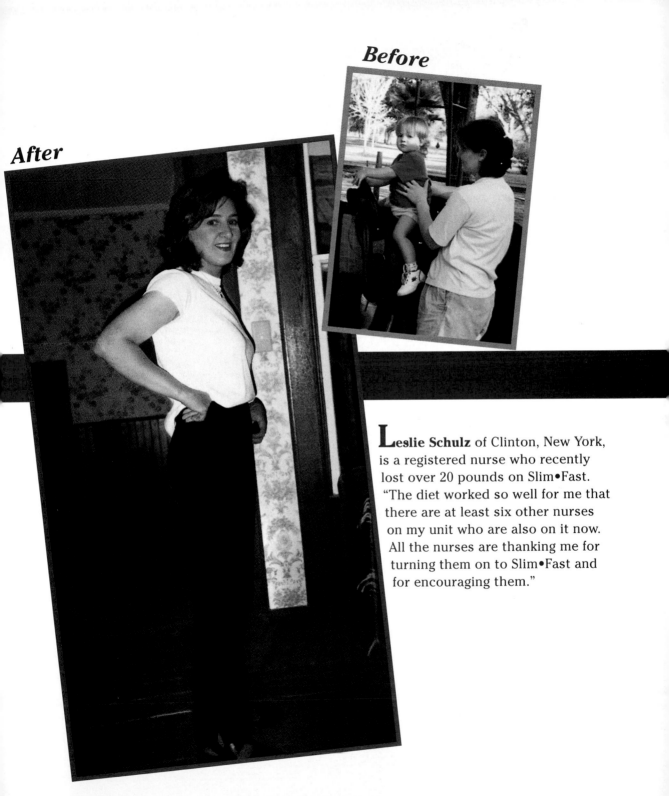

**Before**

**After**

**L**eslie **Schulz** of Clinton, New York, is a registered nurse who recently lost over 20 pounds on Slim•Fast. "The diet worked so well for me that there are at least six other nurses on my unit who are also on it now. All the nurses are thanking me for turning them on to Slim•Fast and for encouraging them."

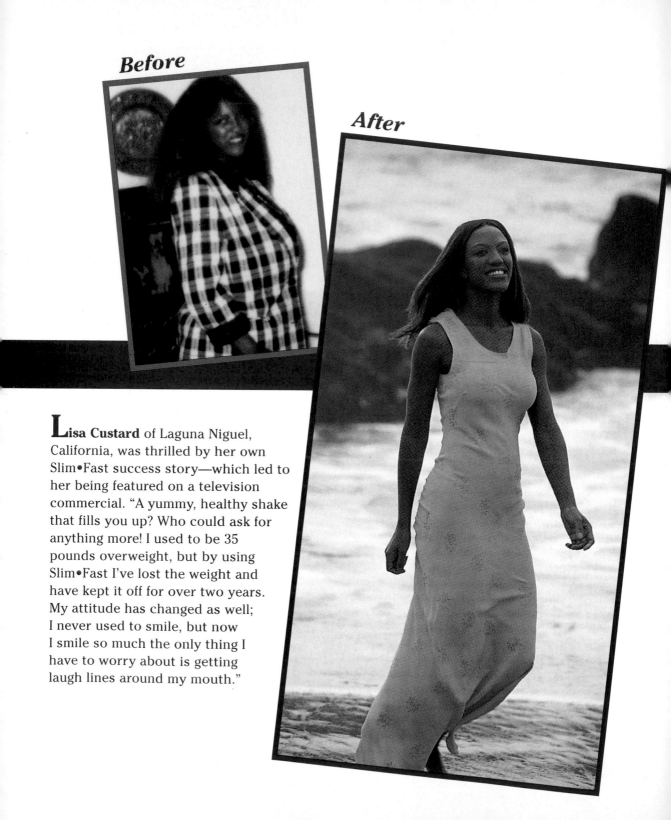

**Before**

**After**

**L**isa **Custard** of Laguna Niguel, California, was thrilled by her own Slim•Fast success story—which led to her being featured on a television commercial. "A yummy, healthy shake that fills you up? Who could ask for anything more! I used to be 35 pounds overweight, but by using Slim•Fast I've lost the weight and have kept it off for over two years. My attitude has changed as well; I never used to smile, but now I smile so much the only thing I have to worry about is getting laugh lines around my mouth."

## Before

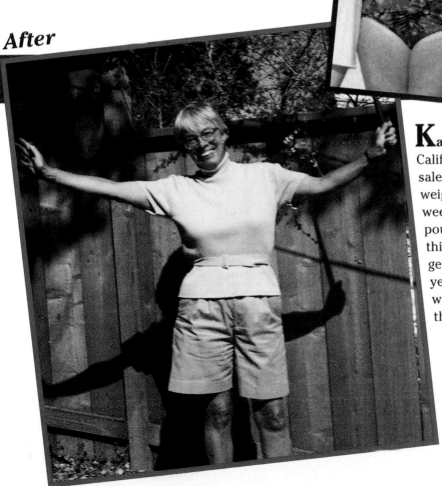

## After

**K**atle Taggart of San Rafael, California, a sixty-year-old saleswoman, reached her weight-loss goal in twelve weeks; she now weighs 35 pounds less than she did at this time last year. "I can get into clothes from seven years ago," she says. "I only wonder why I didn't get with the program much earlier."

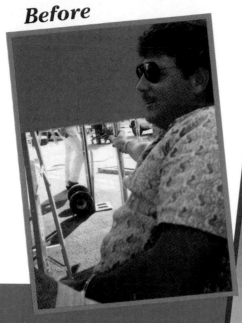

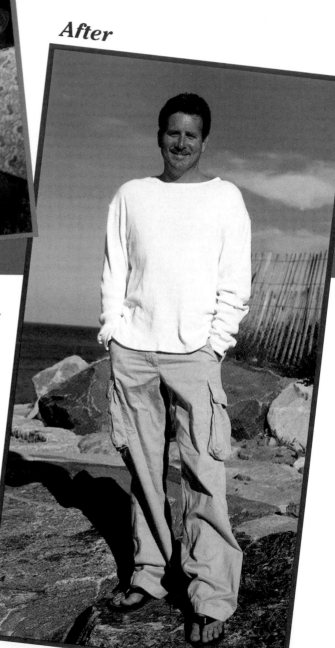

**A**ndy Fisher of Gainesville, Florida, a TV cameraman and diving aficionado, lost 43 pounds on the Slim•Fast Plan—which he discovered while he was shooting Slim•Fast commercials featuring other successful dieters. "When I put on a wet suit," he remembers, "it was a bad situation—I was fat." Today, his life is different. "I'm ecstatic about what I've done for myself. I can't tell you how good I feel—I feel young and rejuvenated. Right now I have the energy to do anything."

**Before**

**After**

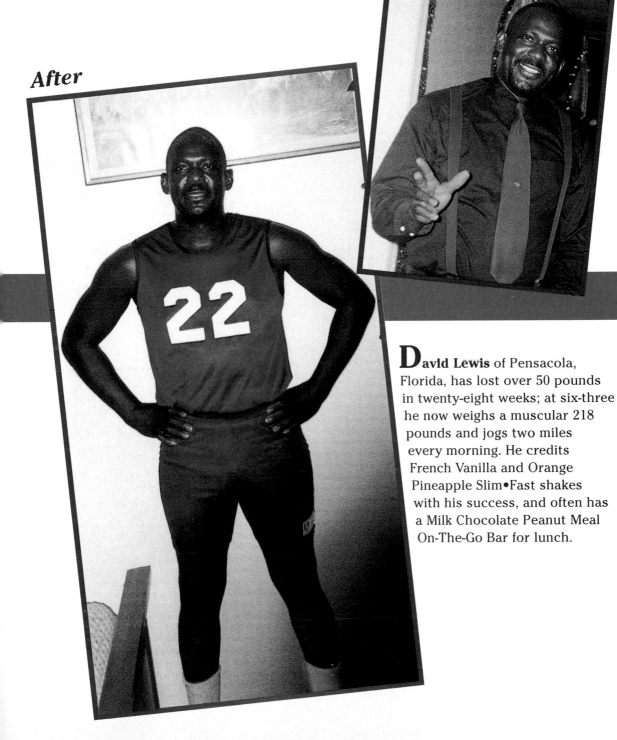

**D**avid Lewis of Pensacola, Florida, has lost over 50 pounds in twenty-eight weeks; at six-three he now weighs a muscular 218 pounds and jogs two miles every morning. He credits French Vanilla and Orange Pineapple Slim•Fast shakes with his success, and often has a Milk Chocolate Peanut Meal On-The-Go Bar for lunch.

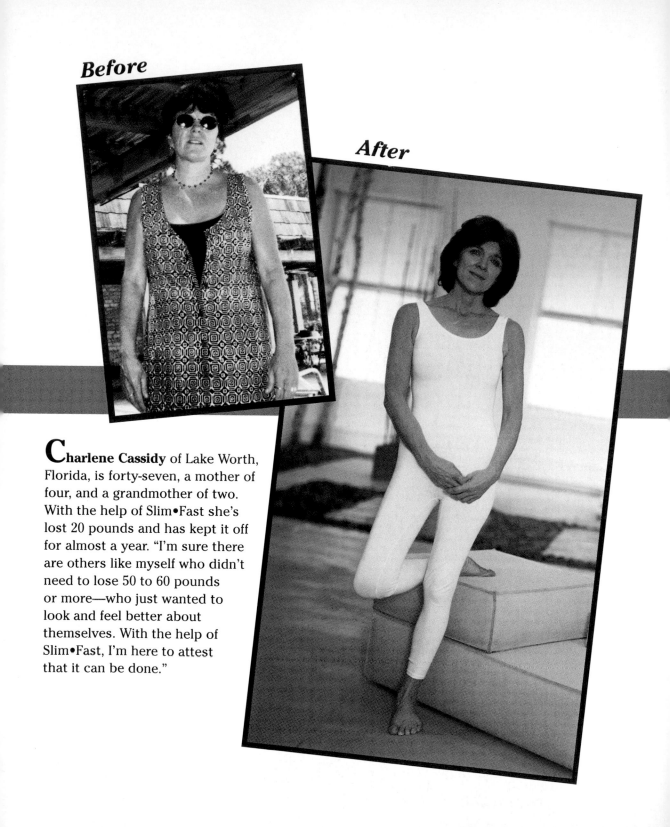

**Before**

**After**

**C**harlene Cassidy of Lake Worth, Florida, is forty-seven, a mother of four, and a grandmother of two. With the help of Slim•Fast she's lost 20 pounds and has kept it off for almost a year. "I'm sure there are others like myself who didn't need to lose 50 to 60 pounds or more—who just wanted to look and feel better about themselves. With the help of Slim•Fast, I'm here to attest that it can be done."

**After**

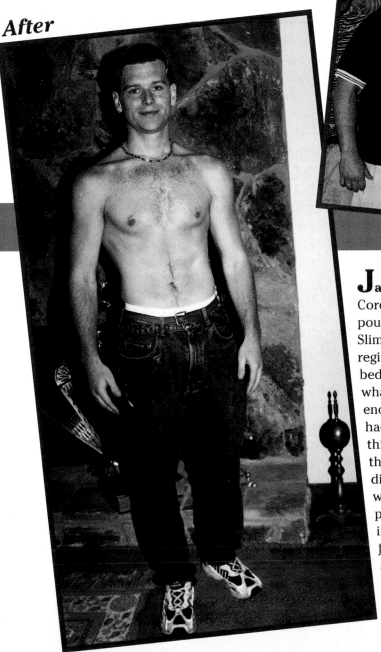

**J**ay **Woodard** of Rancho Cordova, California, lost 100 pounds in less than a year using Slim•Fast and a moderate exercise regimen. "One day when I got out of bed and got on the scale, I weighed what I considered to be an enormous 250 pounds. I knew I had to lose weight, so the first thing I did was to try to change the way I ate. I tried all kinds of different diets and none of them worked at all. I didn't lose a pound in two months of depriving myself of good foods. Then, just as I was ready to give up, I saw a Slim•Fast commercial, and I thought, 'Why not? One more try.' And, as it turned out, one more try was all I needed."

**Before**

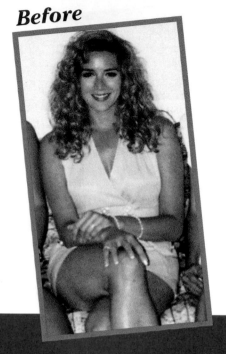

**After**

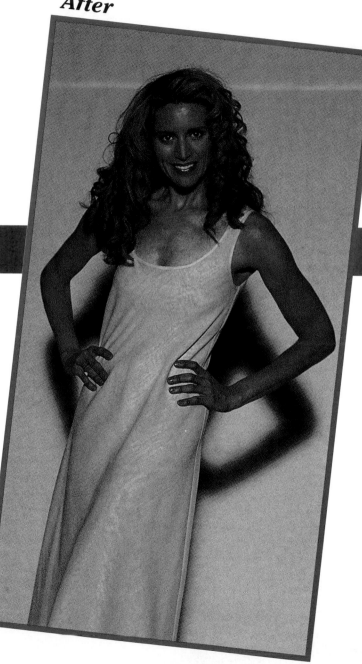

**G**ina **Saadi** of West Hills, California, has three kids, and with all the time she was spending raising them she found she was having a hard time maintaining her ideal weight. "I don't have a minute to eat right," she says. "I gained weight." But after she tried Slim•Fast Meal On-The-Go Bars, she found that she was able to lose the weight she needed—and today she feels more energetic than ever. "I lost 14 pounds on the Slim•Fast Plan," she says. "The peanut butter taste is incredible. It's a well-balanced meal in lots of fantastic flavors. I feel great—I really feel like I have control. It's perfect for my life."

## Before

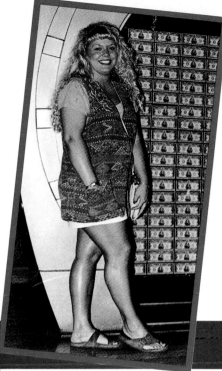

## After in 1996

## ... and in 1999

**D**anna **Warnick** of Richland, Washington, is a twenty-seven-year-old mother of two. "It's a lot harder to keep weight off," she writes, "when you're at home all the time. After the birth of my second child in 1994, I weighed a whopping 200 pounds! I was devastated when I couldn't get it off." Then Danna began the Slim•Fast Plan and found she was able to lose the weight she needed; she now weighs 140 pounds, and has kept the weight off successfully for years. "I feel like a teenager again," she says.

**Before**

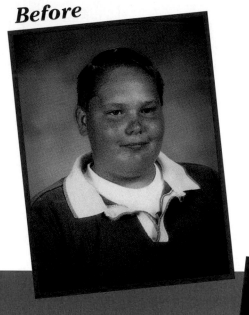

**After**

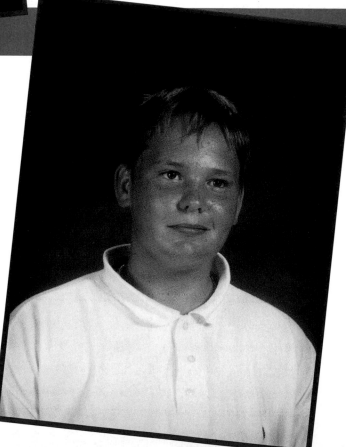

**C**ory Washney of Halifax, Pennyslvania, had such a success story with Slim•Fast that his mother, Beth Ann Lindenmuth, wrote in to rave about her thirteen-year-old son's experience. "My son Cory was up to 244 pounds back in February 1998. He had very little self-esteem and even less energy due to his excessive weight. Finally, I told him about the misery I'd experienced as an overweight child. A few evenings later, he asked me, 'Mom, does Slim•Fast really work?' In three months Cory lost over 25 pounds on the plan; now it's been a year, and with his constant activity he's kept every pound off. Thank you, Slim•Fast, for giving me my energetic, happy boy back!"

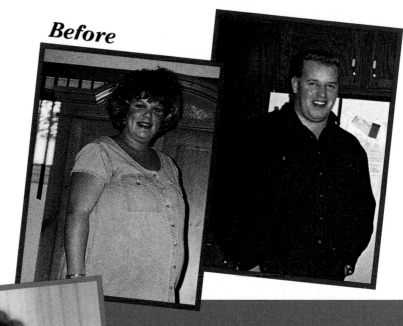

**Before**

**After**

**S**tephanie and Mark Clark of Benton, Illinois, are a tandem Slim•Fast success story. Stephanie gained a lot of weight during her pregnancy in 1995. After the baby was born she had a hard time taking off the weight—until the Slim•Fast Plan helped her lose over 50 pounds in eight and a half months. "I love the taste of Slim•Fast, and it's so filling," she says. "It also curbs my sweet cravings, which I get a lot. I don't have all that much will power, but this is so easy I really don't feel like I'm dieting." Stephanie eventually appeared in a TV commercial for Slim•Fast—which prodded her husband, Mark, to start the program himself. "Everyone was commenting about how great she looked and how I could use some Slim•Fast myself," he says. Mark has lost 65 pounds since 1997, and still brings Meal On-The-Go Bars to work for lunch. "I honestly don't know what Stephanie and I would have done without Slim•Fast."

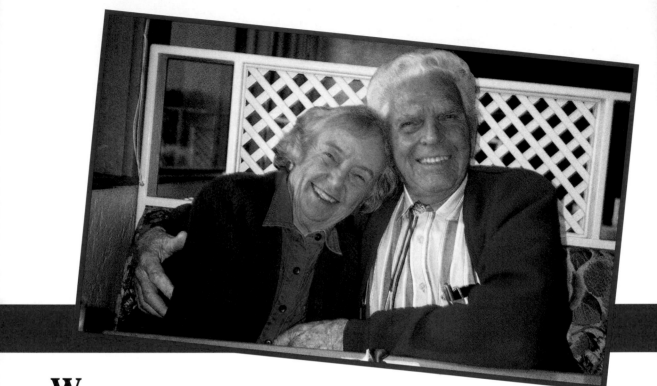

**W**illiam Dale Opperman of Yankton, South
Dakota, has a story that is an inspiration to
dieters young and old: In his late eighties, he
found his weight had increased to 242 pounds,
but in a year's time he managed to reduce to his
goal weight of 165 pounds using the Slim•Fast
Plan. With modest exercise and two shakes a
day, "the whole plan worked so well that I ended
up at the end of the year at the weight I had
promised myself, with hardly any loose skin."
Although he's lost twelve inches from his
waistline, Opperman, now eighty-nine, still uses
all his old belts. "They remind me every day of
what I've accomplished."

example) resets your body's clocks, and can result in symptoms that resemble jet lag. (Ever wonder why it's so hard to fall asleep on Sunday night?)

**Don't exercise within three hours of bedtime.** Exercise elevates your body temperature and quickens your pulse; this energy boost can last a few hours and make it harder for you to fall asleep at bedtime.

# Weighing in—*Every Day*

In recent years, the scale has gotten a bad rap: Many obesity experts warned that people had become too obsessed with the bottom-line number on the scale instead of focusing on healthy habits that would help them lose weight naturally.

But the fact is, the scale remains one of the most useful tools we have in the effort to maintain control of our weight. It's cheap to buy, convenient to use—and it doesn't lie. During the 14-Day Plan you should make it a point to weigh yourself every day—and it's a habit you should continue even after finishing the plan. One recent study conducted by the University of Pittsburgh Medical Center found that people who lost an average of 37 pounds and maintained that weight loss for over seven years weighed themselves much more frequently than overweight people whose weight-loss efforts were less successful.

Weighing yourself every day provides an instant way to monitor your efforts. If you see the scale begin to inch up a pound or two, you can immediately cut back on calories or step up your physical activity. You'll be able to set yourself back on track before you find yourself stepping into a larger pair of jeans.

# 4

# THE 14-DAY PLAN: SEE HOW GREAT YOU CAN FEEL IN JUST TWO WEEKS!

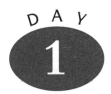

D A Y
1

> *The longest journey is the journey inwards of him who has chosen his destiny, who has started upon his quest for the source of his being.*
>
> —Dag Hammarskjold, former United Nations Secretary General

You are heading off on a journey to a place within yourself where all your good intentions and hopes lie. It's a place you'll visit many times during the next two weeks, as you begin to realize how easy it is to lead a healthy life. You'll be taking hold of your destiny and making a change that will enable you to look better, feel better, and be healthier. Why not do something nice for yourself, to mark the beginning of the journey? Buy yourself a new plant, for example; as you water it and watch it grow, you'll be reminded of how you're nurturing yourself in much the same way.

## DAILY MENU

NOTE: The meals on each day of the plans are interchangeable. If you like some foods better than others, feel free to mix and match: have the dinner from Day 5 again on Day 9, or have one of the dinners for lunch and enjoy a shake when you get home. Just make sure that two of your meals are Slim•Fast shakes or Meal On-The-Go Bars, and the third is one of the sensible meals from the plan.

## BREAKFAST

1 Ultra Slim•Fast Vanilla Powder Mix Shake
   (or your favorite Ultra Slim•Fast shake)
Beverage, noncaloric

## MORNING SNACK

8 ounces nonfat yogurt, artificially sweetened
Beverage, noncaloric

## LUNCH

1 Ultra Slim•Fast Ready-to-Drink Shake
Beverage, noncaloric

## AFTERNOON SNACK

1 Ultra Slim•Fast Nutritional Energy Snack Bar
Beverage, noncaloric

## DINNER

### Salad

   4 cups mixed greens
   1/2 cup sliced mushrooms
   1/2 cucumber, peeled and sliced
   2 tablespoons fat-free dressing
6 ounces broiled, sliced turkey breast
2 tablespoons cranberry sauce
1/2 cup steamed peas

½ cup steamed carrots
½ cup steamed broccoli
½ medium baked sweet potato
1 cup diet gelatin with 1 kiwi, sliced
Beverage, noncaloric

**EVENING SNACK**

1 pear
Beverage, noncaloric

**DAY 1**   NUTRITIONAL INFORMATION

| Day Total | Calories | Protein | Carbohydrates | Fat | Fiber | Sodium | Cholesterol | Calcium |
|---|---|---|---|---|---|---|---|---|
| | 1,468 | 99 g | 223 g | 24 g (14%) | 35 g | 1,352 mg | 147 mg | 1,363 mg |

**Exercise Must-Do:** Today, concentrate on getting small bursts of exercise: climb stairs, jump rope, pedal, or run on an exercise machine for *five minutes* twice a day. Choose activities that you can do at a moment's notice, and push hard enough to feel worn out when you're finished. Add two ten-minute brisk walks around the neighborhood in the morning and evening, along with a fifteen-minute walk at lunch, and you've got a forty-five-minute workout—a great start.

**Instant Stress Reliever:** At the end of the day, write down any of the little tensions that got to you during the day. Next to them, make two columns. In the first column, rate (from 1 to 10) how strongly you reacted to each of them while they were happening; in the second column, rate how important they seem to you now, in retrospect. The very act of putting your stress into perspective should help to relax you.

**Daily Weigh-In:** _____ (weight in pounds)

**Workbook Assignment:** Write down how you felt after every meal and snack. Consider your hunger level, energy level, and overall mood. Rate how you were feeling from 1 to 5, with 1 being "dissatisfied" and 5 being "extremely satisfied."

| | | | | | |
|---|---|---|---|---|---|
| Breakfast | 1 | 2 | 3 | 4 | 5 |
| Snack | 1 | 2 | 3 | 4 | 5 |
| Lunch | 1 | 2 | 3 | 4 | 5 |
| Snack | 1 | 2 | 3 | 4 | 5 |
| Dinner | 1 | 2 | 3 | 4 | 5 |
| Evening Snack | 1 | 2 | 3 | 4 | 5 |

What were your energy high points during the day? Did you feel any low points?

_____

_____

_____

What thoughts were running through your head as you began the plan?

_____

_____

_____

How did you feel knowing that you were nourishing your body with nutritious foods?

_____

_____

_____

Did you experience any hunger or food cravings during the day? If yes, how did you deal with them?

_____

_____

_____

Did you feel satisfied after eating the Slim•Fast shakes and snack bars?

_____

_____

_____

What did you find most challenging about the first day?

_____

_____

_____

What did you find easiest?

_____

_____

_____

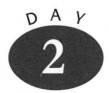

D A Y

2

> *Things do not change; we change.*
>
> —Henry David Thoreau, *Walden*

While you're carefully following this 14-Day Plan, don't forget to take some time to be spontaneous. Plan a family outing with no destination in mind. Just hop in the car and see where you wind up. Let someone else make the plans for the evening and surprise you. Or take a different route home and get a little lost. You'll have an adventure trying to find your way out—and along the way you'll be breaking up your old routine and giving yourself a chance to see life from a new perspective.

## DAILY MENU

### BREAKFAST

1 Ultra Slim•Fast Meal On-The-Go Bar
    (or your favorite Ultra Slim•Fast shake)
4 ounces orange juice
Beverage, noncaloric

### MORNING SNACK

1 apple
Beverage, noncaloric

### LUNCH

1 Ultra Slim•Fast Ready-to-Drink Shake
Beverage, noncaloric

**AFTERNOON SNACK**

## Celery and Carrot Sticks

    1 large carrot, ends removed, peeled, and cut into strips
    1 celery stalk, washed and cut into strips
Beverage, noncaloric

**DINNER**

## Spinach Salad

    4 cups chopped spinach, well-washed
    1/4 cup chopped red onion
    1/2 cup sliced mushrooms
    2 tablespoons fat-free dressing
Savory Broiled Scrod (page 53)
1/2 cup steamed white rice
1 cup steamed zucchini and summer squash
6 steamed asparagus spears
1/2 cup pineapple chunks (in water) with 4 graham cracker squares
Beverage, noncaloric

**EVENING SNACK**

1 Ultra Slim•Fast Energy Snack Bar
Beverage, noncaloric

**DAY 2**   NUTRITIONAL INFORMATION

| Day Total | Calories | Protein | Carbohydrates | Fat | Fiber | Sodium | Cholesterol | Calcium |
|-----------|----------|---------|---------------|-----|-------|--------|-------------|---------|
|  | 1,431 | 73 g | 235 g | 25 g (16%) | 27 g | 1,732 mg | 116 mg | 1,124 mg |

# Savory Broiled Scrod

*Total preparation time: 12 minutes*

½ cup low-calorie mayonnaise

¼ yellow onion, peeled, and grated or very finely diced (substitute 1 tablespoon minced dried onion)

2 tablespoons lemon juice

1¾ pounds scrod fillet (substitute haddock, pollock, or other white fish)

1 large tomato, washed and thinly sliced

1.  Preheat broiler.
2.  In a small mixing bowl, combine mayonnaise with grated onion and lemon juice; mix well.
3.  Rinse fish and pat dry. Place on a flat metal tray or broiler pan. Spoon mayonnaise sauce over fish to cover, and top with sliced tomato. Broil 6 to 7 minutes or until fish flakes easily with a fork or becomes translucent.

SERVES 4

NUTRITIONAL INFORMATION PER SERVING

|  | Calories | Protein | Carbohydrates | Fat | Fiber | Sodium | Cholesterol | Calcium |
|---|---|---|---|---|---|---|---|---|
| **Savory Broiled Scrod** | 263 | 39 g | 8 g | 7 g (25%) | 1 g | 286 mg | 101 mg | 29 mg |

**Exercise Must-Do**: See an opportunity to get yourself moving? Take advantage of it. Help your neighbor bring in a heavy package; park in a space at the far side of the lot and walk; skip the cleaning lady and clean your house yourself; forgo the leaf blower and rake; trade the backyard barbecues for a hike to a picnic spot.

**Instant Stress Reliever**: Sit comfortably and close your eyes. Breathe slowly, becoming aware of the breath passing in and out of your body. Every time you exhale, say the word "Relax" to yourself. As you say it, let the word take effect on the various parts of your body: untense your forehead, loosen your shoulders, relax your arms and legs. Round your back from the waist and reach toward your toes. Come back up and open your eyes.

**Daily Weigh-In:** _____ (weight in pounds)

**Workbook Assignment:** Write down how you felt after every meal and snack. Consider your hunger level, energy level, and overall mood. Rate how you were feeling from 1 to 5, with 1 being "dissatisfied" and 5 being "extremely satisfied."

| | | | | | |
|---|---|---|---|---|---|
| Breakfast | 1 | 2 | 3 | 4 | 5 |
| Snack | 1 | 2 | 3 | 4 | 5 |
| Lunch | 1 | 2 | 3 | 4 | 5 |
| Snack | 1 | 2 | 3 | 4 | 5 |
| Dinner | 1 | 2 | 3 | 4 | 5 |
| Evening Snack | 1 | 2 | 3 | 4 | 5 |

What did you find easier about the second day? Do you feel like you're off to a good start?

_____

_____

_____

How are your friends and family reacting to your decision to go on the plan? Are they encouraging you and supporting your efforts? If not, is there someone else who might be willing to go on the 14-Day Plan with you and serve as your buddy?

_____

_____

_____

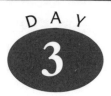

DAY

3

> *Let love, life, and hope be the motivating forces in my thoughts*
> *and acts day by day.*
>
> —Edgar Cayce, therapist and spiritualist

Take ten minutes in the morning to write down one goal that you're setting for yourself today. This should be a character-building goal—the kind of
wish that's usually preceded by words such as "I only wish I could be
more . . ." Today, give yourself permission to act this way—whether it means
taking a little more time with your children or saying "no" to a project you
don't want to do. Give yourself a day to try on your new self. Remember, you
can always slip back into your old self tomorrow.

## DAILY MENU

### BREAKFAST

1 Ultra Slim•Fast Chocolate Royale Powder Shake
    (or your favorite Ultra Slim•Fast shake)
Beverage, noncaloric

### MORNING SNACK

1 orange
Beverage, noncaloric

**LUNCH**

1 Ultra Slim•Fast Meal On-The-Go Bar
15 grapes
Beverage, noncaloric

**AFTERNOON SNACK**

1 Ultra Slim•Fast Nutritional Energy Snack Bar
Beverage, noncaloric

**DINNER**

1 cup low-fat lentil soup (commercially prepared)
Whole Wheat Pasta with Spinach Pesto (page 58)
Baked Golden Acorn Squash (page 59)
½ cup steamed green beans
⅛ honeydew melon
Beverage, noncaloric

**EVENING SNACK**

1 medium banana
Beverage, noncaloric

**DAY 3**   NUTRITIONAL INFORMATION

| Day Total | Calories | Protein | Carbohydrates | Fat | Fiber | Sodium | Cholesterol | Calcium |
|---|---|---|---|---|---|---|---|---|
| | 1,478 | 61 g | 269 g | 26 g (16%) | 46 g | 1,072 mg | 31 mg | 1,480 mg |

# Whole Wheat Pasta with Spinach Pesto

*Total preparation time: 15 minutes*

4 ounces whole wheat pasta (you may also substitute sun-dried tomato
    pasta)

$1/2$ pound fresh spinach, stems removed, rinsed well, and shredded

2 cloves garlic, peeled and minced

$1/4$ cup pine nuts

$1/2$ cup grated Parmesan cheese

1 cup plain nonfat yogurt

1 tablespoon olive oil

1. Set a large saucepan of water to boil. Cook pasta according to package
   directions until barely tender to bite. Drain, cover, and keep warm.
2. Meanwhile, prepare the pesto: In a blender or food processor, combine
   spinach, garlic, pine nuts, Parmesan cheese, yogurt, and olive oil. Blend
   or whirl until pureed.
3. Place cooked pasta in a large shallow serving bowl, top with pesto, and
   mix thoroughly.

SERVES 4

NUTRITIONAL INFORMATION PER SERVING

| | Calories | Protein | Carbohydrates | Fat | Fiber | Sodium | Cholesterol | Calcium |
|---|---|---|---|---|---|---|---|---|
| Whole Wheat Pasta with Spinach Pesto | 364 | 19 g | 50 g | 12 g (30%) | 8 g | 288 mg | 11 mg | 295 mg |

# Baked Golden Acorn Squash

*Total preparation time: 65 minutes*

Vegetable cooking spray
2 medium acorn squash, halved, seeds removed, and rinsed
2 tablespoons maple syrup
1/2 teaspoon ground cinnamon
1 packet artificial sweetener or 1/2 teaspoon loose artificial sweetener
1/4 teaspoon ground black pepper

1.  Preheat oven to 350°F.
2.  Spray a 9 x 13-inch baking pan with vegetable cooking spray. Lay squash halves, cut side down, in the baking pan. Bake, uncovered, until tender when pierced with a fork, 45 minutes.
3.  Turn squash halves cut side up. Drizzle maple syrup over squash and sprinkle with cinnamon, sweetener, and black pepper. Continue baking until edges are browned, 15 minutes.

SERVES 4

NUTRITIONAL INFORMATION PER SERVING

|  | Calories | Protein | Carbohydrates | Fat | Fiber | Sodium | Cholesterol | Calcium |
|---|---|---|---|---|---|---|---|---|
| **Baked Golden Acorn Squash** | 113 | 2 g | 30 g | 0.2 g (2%) | 3 g | 7 mg | 0 mg | 82 mg |

**Exercise Must-Do:** Use some TV time to tone and strengthen your abdominal muscles and chest, by doing some crunches and modified pushups.

*To do a crunch,* lie on your back with your knees bent and your arms crossed over your chest. While keeping your eyes on your knees, inhale and raise your shoulders and back a couple of inches off the floor. Exhale and lower back to the floor. Do as many as you can.

*For a modified pushup,* position yourself on your hands and knees, feet up and crossed at the ankles. Place your hands a bit wider apart than your shoulders; keep your arms straight, but don't lock the elbows. Your neck, back, and waist should be in a straight line. Pull in your abdominal muscles, and slowly lower yourself down until your arms are bent 90 degrees, exhaling as you go. Inhale while pushing yourself up. Do a set of ten, or as many as you can.

**Instant Stress Reliever**: Try giving yourself an aromatherapy oil treatment—a deep conditioning treatment to soften your hair and your mood. Wet your hair and towel it dry until it's lightly damp. In the palm of your hand blend one to three teaspoons of olive oil (more for longer hair, less for shorter) with a few drops of scented lavender or jasmine oil. Massage the mixture into your scalp, working in small circles from your forehead to the base of your neck. Cover your hair with a plastic bag and wrap a towel around that. Relax for twenty minutes. Put your feet up, listen to your favorite CD, and drink a cup of herbal tea. Shampoo hair thoroughly and rinse clean.

**Daily Weigh-In:** _____ (weight in pounds)

**Workbook Assignment**: Write down how you felt after every meal and snack. Consider your hunger level, energy level, and overall mood. Rate how you were feeling from 1 to 5, with 1 being "dissatisfied" and 5 being "extremely satisfied."

| | | | | | |
|---|---|---|---|---|---|
| Breakfast | 1 | 2 | 3 | 4 | 5 |
| Snack | 1 | 2 | 3 | 4 | 5 |
| Lunch | 1 | 2 | 3 | 4 | 5 |
| Snack | 1 | 2 | 3 | 4 | 5 |
| Dinner | 1 | 2 | 3 | 4 | 5 |
| Evening Snack | 1 | 2 | 3 | 4 | 5 |

Do you sometimes turn to food when you are down or nervous? Do you rely on it for emotional support?

_____

_____

_____

Which emotions tend to work against you when you're trying to lose weight? Anger? Depression? Boredom? PMS? Loneliness? Write down some solutions you've come up with to deal with these emotions in ways other than food.

_____

_____

_____

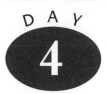

D A Y

**4**

> *Learning to love yourself—it is the greatest love of all.*
> —"The Greatest Love of All,"
> Michael Masser and Linda Cred

Don't hide behind nondescript clothes or hair. Even if you're working on improving your appearance, you should take pride in the way you look right now. Buy yourself a new shirt in the hottest color, or pants cut in a trendy style (even if you may need a smaller size in a few months). Update your hairstyle. Taking care of yourself sends the world a message: I like myself, and others ought to like me, too.

## DAILY MENU

## LUNCHEON MEAL

## BREAKFAST

1 Ultra Slim•Fast Cafe Mocha Powder Shake
    (or your favorite Ultra Slim•Fast shake)
Beverage, noncaloric

## MORNING SNACK

1 Ultra Slim•Fast Nutritional Energy Snack Bar
Beverage, noncaloric

## LUNCH

**Large Tossed Salad**

    2 cups romaine lettuce, washed, dried, and chopped
    2 cups iceberg lettuce, washed, dried, and chopped
    ½ cup sliced mushrooms
    1 tomato, quartered
    2 tablespoons fat-free dressing
Fancy Turkey Salad (page 64)
One 6-inch round (1½ ounces) pita bread
15 seedless grapes
Beverage, noncaloric

## AFTERNOON SNACK

8 ounces nonfat yogurt, artificially sweetened
Beverage, noncaloric

## DINNER

1 Ultra Slim•Fast Ready-to-Drink Shake
10 baby carrots
2 plums
Beverage, noncaloric

## EVENING SNACK

6 ounces cranberry juice with 4 ounces lime seltzer
Beverage, noncaloric

**DAY 4**   NUTRITIONAL INFORMATION

| Day Total | Calories | Protein | Carbohydrates | Fat | Fiber | Sodium | Cholesterol | Calcium |
|-----------|----------|---------|---------------|-----|-------|--------|-------------|---------|
|           | 1,436    | 99 g    | 227 g         | 18 g (11%) | 25 g | 1,434 mg | 167 mg | 1,575 mg |

# Fancy Turkey Salad

*Total preparation time: 40 minutes*

Vegetable cooking spray
1¾ pounds turkey breast tenders *or* 1½ pounds leftover cooked turkey
   breast
2 tablespoons plain nonfat yogurt
2 teaspoons lemon juice
1 tablespoon low-fat mayonnaise
¼ teaspoon onion powder
Dash ground white pepper
2 stalks celery, trimmed, washed, and diced
¼ cup walnuts, chopped
1 medium apple, washed, cored, and diced
1 head red-leaf lettuce, outer leaves removed, washed, dried, and torn into
   bite-size pieces

1. Spray a large nonstick skillet with vegetable cooking spray and heat over medium-high flame. Add turkey and sauté, turning frequently, until cooked through, 6 to 8 minutes (turkey is done when juices run clear or internal temperature is 170°F).

2. Set cooked turkey on platter, cover, and refrigerate to cool, 10 to 15 minutes.

3. Meanwhile, in a small mixing bowl, combine yogurt, lemon juice, mayonnaise, onion powder, and white pepper. Mix with spoon or whisk until blended.

4. When cool, cut cooked turkey into 1-inch cubes and place in a large mixing bowl. Add diced celery, chopped walnuts, and diced apple, fold in the dressing, and gently mix well. Cover and chill in refrigerator 10 to 15 minutes.

5. Place lettuce leaves on 4 salad plates, and top with dressed turkey salad.

SERVES 4

NUTRITIONAL INFORMATION PER SERVING

| | Calories | Protein | Carbohydrates | Fat | Fiber | Sodium | Cholesterol | Calcium |
|---|---|---|---|---|---|---|---|---|
| **Fancy Turkey Salad** | 320 | 54 g | 10 g | 7 g (18%) | 2 g | 140 mg | 142 mg | 62 mg |

**Exercise Must-Do:** Take a twenty-minute power walk, which burns more calories than regular walking and helps improve your fitness. Walk in short quick strides at a pace that's just below a jog. Pump your arms to work your upper body and increase your calorie burn even more.

**Instant Stress Reliever:** Try "Bellow's Breath," a yoga breathing exercise: Exhale for twenty breaths. Take one final deep breath and then breathe comfortably, focusing on your breathing.

**Daily Weigh-In:** _____ (weight in pounds)

**Workbook Assignment:** Write down how you felt after every meal and snack. Consider your hunger level, energy level, and overall mood. Rate how you were feeling from 1 to 5, with 1 being "dissatisfied" and 5 being "extremely satisfied."

| | | | | | |
|---|---|---|---|---|---|
| Breakfast | 1 | 2 | 3 | 4 | 5 |
| Snack | 1 | 2 | 3 | 4 | 5 |
| Lunch | 1 | 2 | 3 | 4 | 5 |
| Snack | 1 | 2 | 3 | 4 | 5 |
| Dinner | 1 | 2 | 3 | 4 | 5 |
| Evening Snack | 1 | 2 | 3 | 4 | 5 |

Spend some time thinking about who is responsible for your weight and why. What issues caused you to be overweight?

_____

_____

_____

Make a list of times when you've blamed someone else for certain situations. Now think of ways in which you could have reclaimed responsibility in those situations.

_____

_____

_____

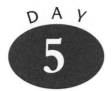

*Many of us become our own worst enemies by holding unrealistic or unduly negative visions of our physical selves.*
—Judith Rodin, Ph.D., *Body Traps*

Chances are you're overestimating your body size. Researchers from the University of South Florida have found that the vast majority of women believe their bodies are 25 percent larger than they actually are. The more inaccurate women are about their body size, the worse they feel about themselves.

Here's a simple technique that might help you see your body the way it really is. Unravel a ball of string, and make a loop that you think reflects the circumference of your waist. Set that aside. Take another piece of string, and make a loop that you think reflects the circumference of your hips. Set that loop aside. Now take two more pieces of string and measure the real circumference of your waist and hips. Compare the length of the real measurements with the loops you estimated for your waist and hips. See the difference?

**DAILY MENU**

**BREAKFAST**

1 Ultra Slim•Fast Cappuccino Delight
    (or your favorite Ultra Slim•Fast shake)
Beverage, noncaloric

**MORNING SNACK**

1 tangerine
Beverage, noncaloric

**LUNCH**

1 Ultra Slim•Fast Ready-to-Drink Shake
Beverage, noncaloric

**AFTERNOON SNACK**

1 Ultra Slim•Fast Nutritional Energy Snack Bar
Beverage, noncaloric

**DINNER**

4 ounces tomato juice
"Good-for-You" Fried Chicken (page 69)
**Rice and Beans**
    1/2 cup steamed brown rice
    1/4 cup canned black beans
    1/2 cup steamed carrots
    1/2 cup steamed spinach
1 nectarine (sliced) with 2 tablespoons light whipped topping
Beverage, noncaloric

**EVENING SNACK**

3 cups plain air-popped popcorn
Beverage, noncaloric

**DAY 5**   NUTRITIONAL INFORMATION

| Day Total | Calories | Protein | Carbohydrates | Fat | Fiber | Sodium | Cholesterol | Calcium |
|---|---|---|---|---|---|---|---|---|
| | 1,425 | 91 g | 204 g | 29 g (18%) | 31 g | 1,230 mg | 162 mg | 1,233 mg |

# "Good–for–You" Fried Chicken

*Total preparation time: 15 minutes*

1¾ **pounds boneless, skinless chicken breasts**
½ **teaspoon paprika**
¼ **teaspoon salt**
½ **teaspoon ground black pepper**
¼ **cup wheat germ**
2 **teaspoons olive oil**

1. Rinse chicken and pat dry. With a mallet or meat tenderizer, lightly pound until each breast is ⅓ to ½ inch thick.
2. On a plate, thoroughly mix paprika, salt, pepper, and wheat germ. Dip each piece of chicken in the spice mixture to coat evenly, and set aside.
3. Heat the oil in a large nonstick pan over medium-high heat. Add the chicken breasts and sauté 2 to 3 minutes on each side, until lightly brown and juices run clear when pricked with a fork, or internal temperature is 170°F. Remove from pan and serve immediately.

SERVES 4

NUTRITIONAL INFORMATION PER SERVING

|  | Calories | Protein | Carbohydrates | Fat | Fiber | Sodium | Cholesterol | Calcium |
|---|---|---|---|---|---|---|---|---|
| **"Good-for-You" Fried Chicken** | 383 | 53 g | 4 g | 16 g (38%) | 1 g | 267 mg | 143 mg | 29 mg |

**Exercise Must-Do:** Today, work on increasing your flexibility. Whether you're off for a short hike or a long jog, here's a stretch you should do beforehand to loosen up your hamstrings and help prevent injury: Stand and place a chair in front of you. Put one heel on the chair, with the leg extended; lean forward from the hips until you feel gentle resistance. Hold for 30 seconds. Repeat on the other leg.

**Instant Stress Reliever:** One good way to release all the stress and tension stored in your muscles is by practicing progressive muscle relaxation. Lie back comfortably and close your eyes. Working your way from your toes to your head, tense each muscle group for two seconds and then release. Curl your toes, hold for two seconds, release. Flex your feet, hold for two seconds, release. Tighten your shins, tense your thighs, scrunch your fingers into a fist, tense your arms, shrug your shoulders, curl your back, purse your lips, and tighten your forehead. After you've tensed and released each muscle group, tense them all together and release. Your body should be completely relaxed.

**Daily Weigh-In:** _____ (weight in pounds)

**Workbook Assignment:** Write down how you felt after every meal and snack. Consider your hunger level, energy level, and overall mood. Rate how you were feeling from 1 to 5, with 1 being "dissatisfied" and 5 being "extremely satisfied."

| | | | | | |
|---|---|---|---|---|---|
| Breakfast | 1 | 2 | 3 | 4 | 5 |
| Snack | 1 | 2 | 3 | 4 | 5 |
| Lunch | 1 | 2 | 3 | 4 | 5 |
| Snack | 1 | 2 | 3 | 4 | 5 |
| Dinner | 1 | 2 | 3 | 4 | 5 |
| Evening Snack | 1 | 2 | 3 | 4 | 5 |

Complete the following sentences: I love food because . . .
I hate food because . . .

_____

_____

_____

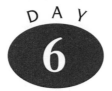

D A Y
6

> *God has not condemned me. No more do I.*
> —Marianne Williamson, *A Course in Miracles*

Today's a day to silence any critical voices that might be rattling around in your head. If you call yourself "thunder thighs" when you're working out, stop. You wouldn't put up with a stranger calling you names, would you? Concentrate on your strengths instead of your perceived shortcomings—it'll help you stay focused on your brilliant future.

**DAILY MENU**

**BREAKFAST**

1 Ultra Slim•Fast Shake, choose your favorite
Beverage, noncaloric

**MORNING SNACK**

1 Ultra Slim•Fast Nutritional Energy Snack Bar
Beverage, noncaloric

**LUNCH**

1 Ultra Slim•Fast Meal On-The-Go Bar
**Celery and Carrot Sticks**
    1 large carrot, ends removed, peeled, and cut into strips
    1 celery stalk, washed and cut into strips
Beverage, noncaloric

**AFTERNOON SNACK**

6 fat-free whole-wheat crackers
Beverage, noncaloric

**DINNER**

Salad

    4 cups green-leaf lettuce, washed, dried, and chopped
    1 tomato, quartered
    ½ cup green bell pepper, washed, cored, and diced
    2 tablespoons balsamic vinegar
6 ounces broiled tuna fillet with lemon and dill
6-inch piece corn on the cob
½ cup baked butternut squash
½ cup steamed green beans
¼ cantaloupe
Beverage, noncaloric

**EVENING SNACK**

1 cup diet gelatin with 1 cup canned peaches in juice
Beverage, noncaloric

**DAY 6**    NUTRITIONAL INFORMATION

| Day Total | Calories | Protein | Carbohydrates | Fat | Fiber | Sodium | Cholesterol | Calcium |
|---|---|---|---|---|---|---|---|---|
| | 1,451 | 92 g | 230 g | 24 g (15%) | 38 g | 809 mg | 103 mg | 1,209 mg |

**Exercise Must-Do:** Do a set of butt-lifters—a quick toning move—at your desk at work. First, with feet together, stand behind a chair and hold on to the back. Lunge back with your right leg, placing the ball of your right foot on the floor. Then, lower the right knee until the left thigh is almost parallel to the floor. Keep the left knee in line above the ankle—don't lean forward. Then return to the starting position. Do 15 repetitions, then repeat on the other leg.

**Instant Stress Reliever**: Here's another easy yoga pose: the cross-legged forward bend. On the floor, sit tall with legs crossed between ankles and shins. Press your fingers into the floor behind you for support. Lengthen your waist and lift your chest. Hold for a minute. Take long, deep breaths, expanding your belly on each inhale, pulling your navel in on each exhale. On an exhale, slowly release torso forward, bending from hips. Rest arms and head on the floor or a pillow. Relax your shoulders and neck, holding for one minute.

**Daily Weigh-In:** _____ (weight in pounds)

**Workbook Assignment**: Write down how you felt after every meal and snack. Consider your hunger level, energy level, and overall mood. Rate how you were feeling from 1 to 5, with 1 being "dissatisfied" and 5 being "extremely satisfied."

| | | | | | |
|---|---|---|---|---|---|
| Breakfast | 1 | 2 | 3 | 4 | 5 |
| Snack | 1 | 2 | 3 | 4 | 5 |
| Lunch | 1 | 2 | 3 | 4 | 5 |
| Snack | 1 | 2 | 3 | 4 | 5 |
| Dinner | 1 | 2 | 3 | 4 | 5 |
| Evening Snack | 1 | 2 | 3 | 4 | 5 |

What are your trigger foods—the foods that you find most difficult to resist?

_____

_____

_____

When do you tend to binge on them and why?

_____

_____

_____

How has the 14-Day Plan helped you get a handle on your eating habits?

_____

_____

_____

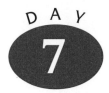

D A Y
7

*You cannot teach a man anything. You can only help him to
find it within himself.*

—Galileo

As you continue with the 14-Day Plan, you're doing everything possible to improve your health by eating right, exercising, and managing stress. While you're making the most out of your life, spend some time thinking about how you deal with life's little snags. Do you have trouble rolling with the punches when things don't go as expected? Consider finding other ways to cope with trials when they occur.

**DAILY MENU**

**BREAKFAST**

1 Ultra Slim•Fast Strawberry Powder Mix
    (or your favorite Ultra Slim•Fast shake)
Beverage, noncaloric

**MORNING SNACK**

1 pear
Beverage, noncaloric

**LUNCH**

1 Ultra Slim•Fast Ready-to-Drink Shake
1 cup strawberries
Beverage, noncaloric

**AFTERNOON SNACK**

1/2 bagel (3 ounces) with 1 tablespoon fat-free cream cheese
Beverage, noncaloric

**DINNER OUT (SUGGESTIONS)**

**Tossed Salad**

    2 cups romaine, washed, dried, and chopped
    2 cups iceberg lettuce, washed, dried, and chopped
    6 cherry tomatoes
    1/2 cup sliced mushrooms
6 ounces lean broiled sirloin steak
1/2 baked potato
1 cup steamed broccoli and cauliflower
1/2 cup steamed peas
1/2 cup fruit sorbet with 1 cup strawberries
Beverage, noncaloric

**EVENING SNACK**

1 Ultra Slim•Fast Nutritional Energy Snack Bar
Beverage, noncaloric

**DAY 7**    NUTRITIONAL INFORMATION

| Day Total | Calories | Protein | Carbohydrates | Fat | Fiber | Sodium | Cholesterol | Calcium |
|---|---|---|---|---|---|---|---|---|
| | 1,432 | 97 g | 216 g | 24 g (15%) | 33 g | 1,133 mg | 172 mg | 1,271 mg |

**Exercise Must-Do**: Get a real workout without breaking up your daily routine. Instead of strolling to pick up your children from a friend's house, get a real move on. Take the dog for an extra walk instead of playing fetch. Bike over to work instead of driving.

**Instant Stress Reliever**: Give yourself a soothing salt scrub. Combine two cups of sea salt with half a cup of shower gel in a small bowl until blended. (Don't use table salt; the grains are too small and will melt.) In the shower or bath, splash yourself with warm water and work the salt mixture into your skin using small circular motions. Pay special attention to rough areas like knees, elbows, and the soles of your feet. After covering your body, rinse and lightly towel dry. Apply a lavish coat of skin moisturizer.

**Daily Weigh-In**: _____ (weight in pounds)

**Workbook Assignment**: Write down how you felt after every meal and snack. Consider your hunger level, energy level, and overall mood. Rate how you were feeling from 1 to 5, with 1 being "dissatisfied" and 5 being "extremely satisfied."

| | | | | | |
|---|---|---|---|---|---|
| Breakfast | 1 | 2 | 3 | 4 | 5 |
| Snack | 1 | 2 | 3 | 4 | 5 |
| Lunch | 1 | 2 | 3 | 4 | 5 |
| Snack | 1 | 2 | 3 | 4 | 5 |
| Dinner | 1 | 2 | 3 | 4 | 5 |
| Evening Snack | 1 | 2 | 3 | 4 | 5 |

You've completed the first half of the plan. How do you feel?

_____

_____

_____

What goals of your life do you feel you're about "halfway" toward fulfilling?

_____

_____

_____

What plans do you have for fulfilling them?

_____

_____

_____

D A Y

8

*Discipline is the bridge between goals and achievements.*
—Anonymous

"Happy people are often in a zone called 'flow,' absorbed in a task that challenges them without overwhelming them," observed David Myers, Ph.D., author of *The Pursuit of Happiness*. Today, take at least thirty minutes to challenge your mind by doing something different from your ho-hum routine. Play Scrabble, do a *New York Times* crossword puzzle, practice on an instrument you haven't touched in years, or start a home-improvement project you've been putting off.

## DAILY MENU

### BREAKFAST
1 Ultra Slim•Fast Cafe Mocha Powder Mix
    (or your favorite Ultra Slim•Fast shake)
Beverage, noncaloric

### MORNING SNACK
¾ ounce packet apple chips (or ¾ ounce dried fruit)
1 cup diet hot cocoa
Beverage, noncaloric

## LUNCH

1 Ultra Slim•Fast Meal On-The-Go Bar
**Celery and Carrot Sticks with Salsa**
    1 celery stalk, washed and cut into strips
    1 large carrot, ends removed, peeled, and cut into strips
    ½ cup salsa
Beverage, noncaloric

## AFTERNOON SNACK

1 Ultra Slim•Fast Nutritional Energy Snack Bar
Beverage, noncaloric

## DINNER

1 cup canned low-fat vegetable soup
Salad Niçoise (recipe below)
1 ounce whole wheat roll
¼ cantaloupe
Beverage, noncaloric

## EVENING SNACK

1 banana
Beverage, noncaloric

**DAY 8**   NUTRITIONAL INFORMATION

| Day Total | Calories | Protein | Carbohydrates | Fat | Fiber | Sodium | Cholesterol | Calcium |
|---|---|---|---|---|---|---|---|---|
| | 1,490 | 79 g | 243 g | 24 g (14%) | 30 g | 2,521 mg | 65 mg | 2,222 mg |

# Salade Niçoise

*Total preparation time: 25 minutes*

1 pound new potatoes, scrubbed, peeled, and quartered
1 pound string beans, ends removed and washed
1 head Bibb or Boston lettuce, rinsed, dried, and torn into bite-size pieces
Two 6-ounce cans water-packed tuna, drained and broken into large chunks
One 6-ounce can small black olives, pitted and drained
2 medium tomatoes, washed and cut into wedges

½ pound fat-free cheddar cheese, cut into 1-inch cubes

8 medium button mushrooms, stems removed, washed, and quartered

One 6-ounce jar pimientos, cut into thin strips

¼ cup balsamic vinegar

1.  In a large saucepan, bring 2 quarts water to a boil. Add potatoes, reduce heat to medium, and cook 20 minutes, until fork-tender but firm. Drain and set aside. When cool enough to handle, cut into 1-inch cubes.
2.  Meanwhile, bring another 1 quart water to boil. Add string beans and cook 45 seconds. Drain immediately and rinse under cold water to preserve color.
3.  Arrange the salad: Divide lettuce among 4 plates, and top with even divisions of potatoes, string beans, tuna, olives, tomatoes, cheese, mushrooms, and pimientos. Top each serving with 2 tablespoons balsamic vinegar.

SERVES 4

NUTRITIONAL INFORMATION PER SERVING

|  | Calories | Protein | Carbohydrates | Fat | Fiber | Sodium | Cholesterol | Calcium |
|---|---|---|---|---|---|---|---|---|
| **Salade Niçoise** | 430 | 43 g | 44 g | 8 g (17%) | 6.5 g | 952 mg | 46 mg | 913 mg |

**Exercise Must-Do:** Practice good posture; over the years, poor posture can take a major toll on your back. The very act of standing up straight can balance your body and help maintain the strength of your spine. What's more, you'll look about five pounds lighter than when you slouch.

*When standing,* tuck in your chin. Keep your back straight and chest held high, shoulders back and relaxed. Keep your stomach and buttocks muscles tight. Keep your knees straight but not locked, and your feet parallel.

*When sitting,* rest your feet flat on the floor, your knees level with your hips. Your middle and lower back should be lightly supported by the back of your chair.

**Instant Stress Reliever:** Let some calming scents take you away from it all. If you need some romance and relaxation, buy yourself a bouquet of flowers that includes lavender, and inhale deeply. If you feel tense or agitated, light a vanilla candle or rub on some vanilla-scented body lotion. If stress is distracting you from doing what you need to do, spray a mint, eucalyptus, or citrus body mist for a mental boost.

**Daily Weigh-In:** _____ (weight in pounds)

**Workbook Assignment:** Write down how you felt after every meal and snack. Consider your hunger level, energy level, and overall mood. Rate how you were feeling from 1 to 5, with 1 being "dissatisfied" and 5 being "extremely satisfied."

| | | | | | |
|---|---|---|---|---|---|
| Breakfast | 1 | 2 | 3 | 4 | 5 |
| Snack | 1 | 2 | 3 | 4 | 5 |
| Lunch | 1 | 2 | 3 | 4 | 5 |
| Snack | 1 | 2 | 3 | 4 | 5 |
| Dinner | 1 | 2 | 3 | 4 | 5 |
| Evening Snack | 1 | 2 | 3 | 4 | 5 |

Describe how you felt about your appearance as a child and teenager. Describe any times when you felt socially rejected because of how you looked.

_____

_____

_____

Describe your feelings about your appearance as an adult. How did you make peace with the physical shortcomings that bothered you as a child?

_____

_____

_____

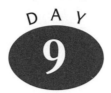

D A Y
9

> *The only motivation I need to write a musical is a phone call*
> *from the producer.*
>
> —Cole Porter

Be your own motivator. Buy a new calendar and use it to chronicle your health and fitness progress. Use a blue marker to check off the days when you eat well and a purple marker to mark the days when you exercise. At the end of every week that you see a lot of color, treat yourself to a small pleasure like a manicure or a new novel. When you don't see a lot of color, redouble your efforts to eat right and exercise.

## DAILY MENU

### BREAKFAST
1 Ultra Slim•Fast Fruit Juice Shake (Powder Mix) with ½ banana
    (or your favorite Ultra Slim•Fast shake)
Beverage, noncaloric

### MORNING SNACK
1 Ultra Slim•Fast Nutritional Energy Snack Bar
Beverage, noncaloric

### LUNCH
1 Ultra Slim•Fast Ready-to-Drink Shake
Beverage, noncaloric

**AFTERNOON SNACK**

¾ ounce pretzels
Beverage, noncaloric

**DINNER**

**Garden Salad**

    4 cups mixed greens, washed and dried
    ½ cucumber, peeled and sliced
    6 cherry tomatoes
    2 tablespoons fat-free dressing
Beef Fajitas (recipe below)
One 10-ounce slice watermelon
Beverage, noncaloric

**EVENING SNACK**

15 grapes
Beverage, noncaloric

**DAY 9**    NUTRITIONAL INFORMATION

| Day Total | Calories | Protein | Carbohydrates | Fat | Fiber | Sodium | Cholesterol | Calcium |
|---|---|---|---|---|---|---|---|---|
| | 1,500 | 87 g | 233 g | 30 g (17%) | 26 g | 1,892 mg | 141 mg | 1,151 mg |

# Beef Fajitas

*Total preparation time: 90 minutes*

    Marinade
        ¼ cup fresh lime juice
        1 medium jalapeño pepper, finely diced
        1 teaspoon cumin
        2 cloves garlic, peeled and minced
        1 tablespoon canola oil
        ½ cup light beer

1¾ pounds lean beef round, 1 to 1½ inches thick

Vegetable cooking spray

2 medium yellow onions, peeled and thinly sliced

2 large green bell peppers, washed, cored, seeded, and cut into ¼-inch
   strips

2 large tomatoes, washed and diced

4 medium low-fat flour or corn tortillas

½ cup salsa

1 cup shredded fat-free Monterey Jack cheese

1. In a shallow glass pan, mix lime juice, jalapeño pepper, cumin, garlic, canola oil, and beer. Add beef; cover and place in refrigerator for 20 minutes (or up to 4 hours), turning once.
2. Preheat oven to 425°F.
3. Transfer the beef to a roasting pan or sheet, and bake 35 to 45 minutes, or until internal temperature is 160°F, for medium. Remove to a platter, cover lightly with aluminum foil, and let stand 15 to 20 minutes (the beef will continue cooking slightly, and will retain its juices). Carve into ¼-inch-thick slices.
4. Meanwhile, heat a large nonstick skillet over high heat and coat lightly with vegetable spray. Add onions and peppers and sauté until wilted, 3 to 4 minutes. Add tomatoes and cook 1 minute more, until heated through. Toss well.
5. Spread the tortillas flat on a large platter. Cover one-third of each tortilla with the sautéed vegetables and top with sliced beef, salsa, and cheese. Roll the tortilla into a tight wrap and let rest 1 minute for the heat of the vegetables to melt the cheese.

SERVES 4

NUTRITIONAL INFORMATION PER SERVING

| | Calories | Protein | Carbohydrates | Fat | Fiber | Sodium | Cholesterol | Calcium |
|---|---|---|---|---|---|---|---|---|
| **Beef Fajitas** | 537 | 57 g | 42 g | 14 g (24%) | 3 g | 702 mg | 126 mg | 268 mg |

**Exercise Must-Do:** Do this twenty-minute circuit-training workout to tone your shoulders, thighs, and arms while giving you a cardiovascular workout. In between each of these three moves, jump rope or run in place for 30 counts. (You'll need a set of dumbbells—3, 5, 10, 15, or 20 pounds, depending on your strength; you can begin by using full soup cans.)

*Shoulder presses.* Grab a set of dumbbells with both hands. Hold the dumbbells slightly above ear level, with palms facing forward and elbows bent at a 90-degree angle. Straighten arms up until almost fully extended. Return to starting position. Do 15 reps.

*Pliés.* Stand with your feet shoulder-width apart, toes pointing slightly out and knees slightly bent. Hold one dumbbell between legs with both hands, and bend your knees until they're at a 90-degree angle, keeping your back straight and your knees in line with your toes. Return to standing position. Do 15 reps.

*Biceps curls.* Stand and hold dumbbells at sides with palms facing forward. Curl the dumbbells up to chest level, then return to starting position. Do 15 reps.

**Instant Stress Reliever:** Too much to do in too little time? Take a new attitude toward time. Turn your attention away from all the things you *have* to do, and focus on one thing that's *not* on your to-do list. Take a moment and really listen to what your children are saying. Try to notice the landscape or interesting buildings when you're driving. Give yourself fifteen minutes a day that are free of interruptions—no phone, TV, or chores—just to be alone with your own thoughts.

**Daily Weigh-In:** _____ (weight in pounds)

**Workbook Assignment:** Write down how you felt after every meal and snack. Consider your hunger level, energy level, and overall mood. Rate how you were feeling from 1 to 5, with 1 being "dissatisfied" and 5 being "extremely satisfied."

| Breakfast | 1 | 2 | 3 | 4 | 5 |
|---|---|---|---|---|---|
| Snack | 1 | 2 | 3 | 4 | 5 |
| Lunch | 1 | 2 | 3 | 4 | 5 |
| Snack | 1 | 2 | 3 | 4 | 5 |
| Dinner | 1 | 2 | 3 | 4 | 5 |
| Evening Snack | 1 | 2 | 3 | 4 | 5 |

Think about any impediments that may be keeping you from exercising. Describe your experiences with exercise as a child.

_____

_____

_____

If you aren't exercising on a regular basis, describe any barriers that you're facing.

_____

_____

_____

Describe some ways you can overcome these barriers.

_____

_____

_____

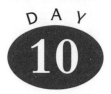

D A Y

10

> *The world is wide, and I will not waste my life in friction when it could be turned into momentum.*
>
> —Frances Willard,
> first leader of the Women's Christian Temperance Union

Start keeping a log of how great you feel as you continue to follow the Slim•Fast Plan. When you have a particularly grueling day (and you feel like you just can't keep up your good health habits), go back and read your log for inspiration.

**DAILY MENU**

**BREAKFAST**
1 Ultra Slim•Fast Meal On-The-Go Bar
    (or your favorite Ultra Slim•Fast shake)
4 ounces orange juice
Beverage, noncaloric

**MORNING SNACK**
1/2 bagel (3 ounces) with 1 tablespoon fat-free cream cheese
Beverage, noncaloric

**LUNCH**
1 Ultra Slim•Fast Chocolate Royale Shake
Beverage, noncaloric

**AFTERNOON SNACK**

1 Ultra Slim•Fast Nutritional Energy Snack Bar
Beverage, noncaloric

**DINNER**

**Spinach Salad**

    4 cups spinach, well-washed, dried, and chopped
    1/2 red onion, peeled and sliced
    4 mushrooms, washed and sliced
    1 hard-cooked egg, peeled and chopped
    2 tablespoons fat-free dressing
Lemon-Garlic Angel Hair (page 90)
1 ounce French bread
**Fruit Salad**
    1/2 cup strawberries
    1/2 cup cubed mango
Beverage, noncaloric

**EVENING SNACK**

1 pear
Beverage, noncaloric

**DAY 10**   NUTRITIONAL INFORMATION

| Day Total | Calories | Protein | Carbohydrates | Fat | Fiber | Sodium | Cholesterol | Calcium |
|---|---|---|---|---|---|---|---|---|
| | 1,450 | 58 g | 240 g | 28 g (17%) | 25 g | 1,883 mg | 242 mg | 1,413 mg |

# Lemon-Garlic Angel Hair

*Total preparation time: 20 minutes*

8 ounces angel hair pasta
1 tablespoon olive oil
4 cloves garlic, peeled and minced
1 cup dry white wine
3 tablespoons lemon juice
One 16-ounce can tomatoes, drained and chopped
1 cup fresh basil, chopped *or* 1 teaspoon dried basil
1/2 cup freshly grated Parmesan cheese
1/4 teaspoon ground black pepper

1. Bring a large pot of water to a boil over high heat. Add pasta and cook according to package directions until al dente. Drain and place in warm serving bowl.
2. Meanwhile, add olive oil and garlic to a large nonstick skillet and cook over medium heat until garlic just begins to brown, about 30 seconds. Remove pan from heat and pour in white wine. Return skillet to medium heat and cook 1 to 2 minutes, until wine is reduced by half. Stir in lemon juice and tomatoes, remove from heat, and set aside.
3. Toss the cooked, drained pasta with the basil, Parmesan cheese, black pepper, and tomato mixture.

SERVES 4

NUTRITIONAL INFORMATION PER SERVING

|  | Calories | Protein | Carbohydrates | Fat | Fiber | Sodium | Cholesterol | Calcium |
|---|---|---|---|---|---|---|---|---|
| Lemon-Garlic Angel Hair | 322 | 14 g | 40 g | 8 g (23%) | 3 g | 441 mg | 10 mg | 236 mg |

**Exercise Must-Do**: Turn a walk in the park into a strength-training workout.

*Take a five-minute warm-up walk.* Find a park bench and do three minutes of *bench pushups* to work your chest, back, arms, and abdominals. Facing a bench seat, place your hands flat on the seat and walk your feet back until your spine, buttocks, and legs are in a straight line and your straightened arms are at a 90-degree angle to the seat. Keeping your abdominal muscles tightened, inhale and bend your arms, lowering yourself down toward the bench. Exhale as you push back up. Aim for 15 to 20 repetitions. Do two sets, resting for 45 seconds between sets.

Next do some *bench step-ups* for about 3 minutes to work your quadriceps (thighs), hamstrings, and buttocks. Stand facing the bench, with your right foot on the seat. Step straight up with your right leg, touching your left foot briefly on the seat for balance. In a slow, controlled motion, step back down until your left foot is flat on the ground. Immediately do the next step-up with the same leg. Do 10 repetitions and repeat on your left leg. Rest for 45 seconds between each leg. Do 2 to 3 sets.

**Instant Stress Reliever**: Enjoy some quiet downtime, and take a moment for some moving meditation. If the weather is nice, take a walk or bike ride outside. If not, use a treadmill or stationary bike or march in place. While you're moving, clear your head of any troubling thoughts and just focus on a thought or word that has personal meaning to you. Keep your mind focused on the movement of your legs, the swinging rhythm of your arms, or the sound of your breath, while letting your mind drift away from any stress or tension.

**Daily Weigh-In:** _____ (weight in pounds)

**Workbook Assignment:** Write down how you felt after every meal and snack. Consider your hunger level, energy level, and overall mood. Rate how you were feeling from 1 to 5, with 1 being "dissatisfied" and 5 being "extremely satisfied."

| | | | | | |
|---|---|---|---|---|---|
| Breakfast | 1 | 2 | 3 | 4 | 5 |
| Snack | 1 | 2 | 3 | 4 | 5 |
| Lunch | 1 | 2 | 3 | 4 | 5 |
| Snack | 1 | 2 | 3 | 4 | 5 |
| Dinner | 1 | 2 | 3 | 4 | 5 |
| Evening Snack | 1 | 2 | 3 | 4 | 5 |

Write down your memories of high-fat and high-sugar food treats that you enjoyed as a child. Did your mother make them especially for you?

_____

_____

_____

Describe your feelings before, during, and after eating a large amount of high-fat food.

_____

_____

_____

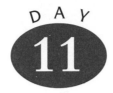

DAY
11

> *We have two ears and one mouth so that we can listen twice as much as we speak.*
>
> —Epictetus

Here's a surprising secret: Even being a better listener can help your makeover along. Good listening creates greater intimacy in relationships, and can even lower blood pressure in people who have hypertension. Try this listening exercise: Sit down with a close friend, family member, or significant other for twenty minutes and express how you each feel about whatever is on your minds. Let one person speak for ten minutes, and make sure the listener doesn't respond—even with facial expressions. Next, reverse roles.

## DAILY MENU

### BREAKFAST

1 Ultra Slim•Fast Rich Chocolate Royale Ready-to-Drink Shake
    (or your favorite Ultra Slim•Fast shake)
Beverage, noncaloric

### MORNING SNACK

2 plums
Beverage, noncaloric

### LUNCH

1 Ultra Slim•Fast Meal On-The-Go Bar
Beverage, noncaloric

## AFTERNOON SNACK

4 ounces fat-free pudding snack
Beverage, noncaloric

## DINNER

### Tomato-Cucumber Salad

    1 large tomato, sliced
    1 cucumber, peeled and sliced
    2 tablespoons fat-free dressing
Mediterranean Leg of Lamb with Roasted Vegetables (page 95)
1/2 cup steamed green beans
1/2 cup sugar-free sorbet
Beverage, noncaloric

## EVENING SNACK

1 Ultra Slim•Fast Nutritional Energy Snack Bar
Beverage, noncaloric

**DAY 11**   NUTRITIONAL INFORMATION

| Day Total | Calories | Protein | Carbohydrates | Fat | Fiber | Sodium | Cholesterol | Calcium |
|-----------|----------|---------|---------------|-----|-------|--------|-------------|---------|
|  | 1,465 | 68 g | 219 g | 37 g (23%) | 24 g | 1,118 mg | 124 mg | 1,109 mg |

# Mediterranean Leg of Lamb with Roasted Vegetables

*Total preparation time: 2 or 2½ hours*

3 cloves garlic, peeled
2 teaspoons freshly ground pepper
½ cup fresh mint, chopped
¼ cup virgin olive oil
2 tablespoons lemon juice
One 5-pound bone-in leg of lamb, trimmed of excess fat
1 pound carrots, tops and bottoms removed, peeled and cut into 2-inch
   pieces
4 large onions, peeled, cut into quarters
4 medium red bliss potatoes

1. Preheat oven to 450°F.
2. In food processor, add garlic, pepper, mint, olive oil, and lemon juice. Pulse to blend, about 30 seconds.
3. Place lamb and marinade in large plastic bag, fastening end with twist tie. Turn bag over several times, thoroughly rubbing marinade over meat. Refrigerate for 30 minutes, or up to two hours.
4. Remove lamb from plastic bag (discard bag). Place lamb in a large roasting pan with rack. Roast, uncovered, for 15 minutes at 450°F. Add carrots, onions, and potatoes to roasting pan, stirring to coat with lamb juices. Reduce oven temperature to 350°F. Roast for approximately 1½ hours, allowing 15 to 20 minutes per pound for average doneness. Check temperature with meat thermometer for desired doneness: For medium, internal temperature should register 145°F, 150°F for medium well.

   Remove lamb to serving platter; cover loosely with foil to keep warm. Let stand for 15 minutes before serving. Surround lamb with vegetables and serve immediately.

SERVES 4, WITH LEFTOVERS

NUTRITIONAL INFORMATION PER SERVING

| | Calories | Protein | Carbohydrates | Fat | Fiber | Sodium | Cholesterol | Calcium |
|---|---|---|---|---|---|---|---|---|
| Mediterranean Leg of Lamb with Roasted Vegetables | 571 | 40 g | 51 g | 24 g (37%) | 8 g | 133 mg | 109 mg | 84 mg |

**Exercise Must-Do**: Finding it hard to get out of bed in the morning? Feeling that afternoon slump? Squeeze in ten minutes of wake-me-up moves. Dance around for five minutes to your favorite CD. Alternate dance moves with knee bends, jumping jacks, and kicks. Spend the next five minutes doing simple stretches. *Stretch #1:* Stand straight and fully extend your arms over your head. Try to touch the ceiling; hold for a count of 5. Repeat two more times. *Stretch #2:* Stand with your feet hip-distance apart, knees slightly bent. Bend at your waist to one side as far as is comfortable. Hold for a count of 5. Bring your torso back to center and repeat, bending to the other side. Do two more repetitions.

**Instant Stress Reliever**: Create an atmosphere that's conducive to a good night's sleep. Use room-darkening shades and a white-noise fan if traffic is keeping you up at night. Sip a cup of chamomile tea just before bed. Spray your pillow with some lavender oil, a natural sleep inducer first used by Cleopatra.

**Daily Weigh-In**: _____ (weight in pounds)

**Workbook Assignment**: Write down how you felt after every meal and snack. Consider your hunger level, energy level, and overall mood. Rate how you were feeling from 1 to 5, with 1 being "dissatisfied" and 5 being "extremely satisfied."

| | | | | | |
|---|---|---|---|---|---|
| Breakfast | 1 | 2 | 3 | 4 | 5 |
| Snack | 1 | 2 | 3 | 4 | 5 |
| Lunch | 1 | 2 | 3 | 4 | 5 |
| Snack | 1 | 2 | 3 | 4 | 5 |
| Dinner | 1 | 2 | 3 | 4 | 5 |
| Evening Snack | 1 | 2 | 3 | 4 | 5 |

Look in the mirror and write down three physical attributes you like best about yourself.

_____

_____

_____

Write down your three strongest personality attributes.

_____

_____

_____

Write down something you accomplished today that you're proud of.

_____

_____

_____

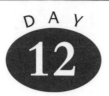

*Every so often it's best to experience yourself as you truly are.*
—Mark Epstein, M.D.,
*Going to Pieces Without Falling Apart*

If you're always expending energy to keep yourself together, looking good, and acting the way you feel you're supposed to, you may wish you could just be *yourself* for a while. Letting go this way can lead to heightened creativity, honesty, and more genuine contact with other people—and yourself.

**DAILY MENU**

**BREAKFAST**

1 Ultra Slim•Fast Vanilla Powder Mix Shake
    (or your favorite Ultra Slim•Fast shake)
Beverage, noncaloric

**MORNING SNACK**

1 Ultra Slim•Fast Nutritional Energy Snack Bar
Beverage, noncaloric

**LUNCH**

1 Ultra Slim•Fast Ready-to-Drink Shake
Beverage, noncaloric

**AFTERNOON SNACK**

½ cup fat-free cottage cheese with ½ cup diced peaches (fresh or canned)
Beverage, noncaloric

**DINNER**

**Tossed Salad**
    4 cups mixed greens
    1 small red onion, peeled and sliced
    ½ cup cooked beets
    2 tablespoons fat-free dressing
Salmon Supreme (page 100)
½ cup steamed green peas
½ cup steamed summer squash
1 cup diet gelatin with 1 kiwi, sliced
Beverage, noncaloric

**EVENING SNACK**

¼ cantaloupe
Beverage, noncaloric

**DAY 12**  NUTRITIONAL INFORMATION

| Day Total | Calories | Protein | Carbohydrates | Fat | Fiber | Sodium | Cholesterol | Calcium |
|---|---|---|---|---|---|---|---|---|
| | 1,440 | 99 g | 217 g | 23 g (14%) | 33 g | 1,778 mg | 142 mg | 1,300 mg |

# Salmon Supreme

*Total preparation time: 25 minutes*

Vegetable cooking spray
4 medium red bliss potatoes, unpeeled, washed, and cut into 1/4-inch slices
Four 7-ounce salmon steaks, about 1 inch thick
2 tablespoons lemon juice
2 tablespoons fat-free cream cheese
1/4 cup fat-free mayonnaise
1/4 teaspoon ground black pepper
2 large carrots, tops and bottom removed, peeled, and grated
2 medium tomatoes, washed and finely diced
1 scallion, trimmed, washed, and finely diced
1/2 lemon, cut into 4 wedges

1. Preheat oven to 400°F. Spray a 9 x 13-inch roasting pan with vegetable spray.
2. Rinse salmon and pat dry. Place potatoes and salmon in a single layer in roasting pan, and drizzle fish with 1 tablespoon lemon juice.
3. In a small bowl, combine remaining tablespoon lemon juice with cream cheese, mayonnaise, and pepper, and mix until smooth. Stir in grated carrots, diced tomatoes, and diced scallion. Top fish and potatoes with vegetable mixture, spreading on top of all.
4. Bake uncovered until potatoes are tender and fish flakes easily to fork, 12 minutes. Preheat broiler. Place under broiler for 60 seconds to brown vegetable mixture. Serve immediately. Garnish with lemon wedges.

SERVES 4

NUTRITIONAL INFORMATION PER SERVING

|  | Calories | Protein | Carbohydrates | Fat | Fiber | Sodium | Cholesterol | Calcium |
|---|---|---|---|---|---|---|---|---|
| Salmon Supreme | 456 | 45 g | 39 g | 13 g (26%) | 4.5 g | 258 mg | 112 mg | 65 mg |

**Exercise Must-Do**: Increase your balance and control with this exercise. Stand with your feet flat directly under your hips, your hands on your hips, and your abs contracted. Bend your right knee, lifting your leg in front of you until your right heel is level with your left knee. With your left hand, press on your right inner thigh, resisting with the muscle. Put your hands back on your hips. Next, keeping hips and shoulders pointing straight ahead and your right foot resting gently on the inside of your left knee, squeeze the muscles in your left leg and pivot your right knee out to the side. Hold for a second, return your knee to the forward-facing position, and lower your foot to the ground. Do 10 reps, alternating sides.

**Instant Stress Reliever**: Practice mindfulness—a heightened state of alertness that will put you more in touch with the world around you. Notice a pen's shape, color, weight, and feel. Sip a cup of warm peppermint tea, focusing on the heat of the liquid and the smell of the mint. Savor a single strawberry and feel its juices wet your tongue. Mindfulness leads to relaxation.

**Daily Weigh-In**: _____ (weight in pounds)

**Workbook Assignment**: Write down how you felt after every meal and snack. Consider your hunger level, energy level, and overall mood. Rate how you were feeling from 1 to 5, with 1 being "dissatisfied" and 5 being "extremely satisfied."

| | | | | | |
|---|---|---|---|---|---|
| Breakfast | 1 | 2 | 3 | 4 | 5 |
| Snack | 1 | 2 | 3 | 4 | 5 |
| Lunch | 1 | 2 | 3 | 4 | 5 |
| Snack | 1 | 2 | 3 | 4 | 5 |
| Dinner | 1 | 2 | 3 | 4 | 5 |
| Evening Snack | 1 | 2 | 3 | 4 | 5 |

Describe the highs and lows in your weight history.

_____

_____

_____

What was your life like when you were heavier? Thinner?

_____

_____

_____

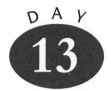

D A Y
13

> *The greater the obstacle, the more glory in overcoming it.*
> —**Molière**

Don't shy away from taking on a project with a heavy workload because you think it will make you stressed and unhappy. Researchers from Ohio State University have found that people who work long hours because they're trying to achieve a goal they've set for themselves—as opposed to working under extreme pressure from above—are usually happy about the work they're doing. So pursue your lofty goals, and look forward to your accomplishments!

**DAILY MENU**

**BREAKFAST**
1 Ultra Slim•Fast Chocolate Royale Powder Mix Shake
   (or your favorite Ultra Slim•Fast shake)
Beverage, noncaloric

**MORNING SNACK**
4 ounces canned fruit (snack pack)
Beverage, noncaloric

**LUNCH**
1 Ultra Slim•Fast Ready-to-Drink Shake
15 baby carrots
Beverage, noncaloric

**AFTERNOON SNACK**

1 Ultra Slim•Fast Nutritional Energy Snack Bar
Beverage, noncaloric

**DINNER**

**Black Bean Salad**
     3/4 cup canned black beans, drained
     1/2 cup red pepper, washed, cored, and diced
     1/4 cup diced onion
     2 tablespoons balsamic vinegar
     6 lettuce leaves
Chicken Stir-Fry over White Rice (page 105)
1/2 cup canned pineapple chunks (water-packed)
Beverage, noncaloric

**EVENING SNACK**

3 cups air-popped popcorn with calorie-free buttery spray
Beverage, noncaloric

**DAY 13**   NUTRITIONAL INFORMATION

| Day Total | Calories | Protein | Carbohydrates | Fat | Fiber | Sodium | Cholesterol | Calcium |
|---|---|---|---|---|---|---|---|---|
| | 1,507 | 85 g | 244 g | 27 g (16%) | 40 g | 1,426 mg | 130 mg | 982 mg |

# Chicken Stir-Fry over White Rice

*Total preparation time: 40 minutes*

1 cup white rice
1 tablespoon olive oil
3 cloves garlic, peeled and minced
1¾ pounds boneless chicken breasts, sliced into strips
1 tablespoon light (reduced-sodium) soy sauce
¼ cup low-sodium chicken broth
1 teaspoon ground ginger
½ teaspoon celery seed
1 pound broccoli, tough stems removed, washed, and cut into flowerets
1 pound carrots, ends removed, peeled, and cut into ½-inch slices
1 pound mushrooms, washed, dried, and sliced
1 medium green pepper, washed, cored, seeded, and cut into strips
1 medium red sweet pepper, washed, cored, seeded, and cut into strips

1. In a medium saucepan, combine rice with 2 cups water and bring to a boil. Immediately reduce heat to very low, cover, and simmer 20 minutes. Turn off flame, and let sit 5 to 10 minutes; fluff with a fork before serving.
2. While the rice is cooking, heat the oil in a wok or large skillet over medium-high flame. Sauté garlic until golden, 30 to 60 seconds. Add chicken and sauté, turning frequently, 5 to 7 minutes or until cooked throughout. Remove chicken from skillet and set aside.
3. In a small bowl, mix soy sauce, broth, ginger, celery seed, and vegetables. Sauté in the same skillet over medium heat until vegetables are tender but still crisp, 3 to 4 minutes. Return chicken to mixture and mix well. Serve immediately over hot white rice.

SERVES 4

NUTRITIONAL INFORMATION PER SERVING

| | Calories | Protein | Carbohydrates | Fat | Fiber | Sodium | Cholesterol | Calcium |
|---|---|---|---|---|---|---|---|---|
| **Chicken Stir-Fry over White Rice** | 598 | 52 g | 61 g | 16 g (24%) | 8 g | 327 mg | 120 mg | 117 mg |

**Exercise Must-Do:** Maximize your walking technique to help you burn more calories without burning yourself out.

• While walking, keep your eyes focused on a spot ten feet in front of you instead of looking at the ground.

• Clench your hands into loose fists and swing them without crossing them (which would twist your torso and slow you down).

• Maintain a short, quick, efficient stride by letting your foot land practically beneath you. Don't step out, but keep more of your stride length behind your body, not in front of it.

• Keep your back straight, neck and shoulders relaxed.

• To soften your landing, try to touch the ground heel first with your ankle flexed, then roll forward to the front of your foot. Push off with flexed toes for your next step.

**Instant Stress Reliever:** The Chinese have developed a series of exercises that promote the flow of *chi*, the life force that flows through the body and regulates its functions.

• Stand with your feet shoulder-width apart and parallel. Bend your knees to a quarter-squat position (about 45 degrees) while keeping your upper body straight. Observe your breathing for a couple of breaths.

• Inhale and bring your arms slowly up in front of you to shoulder height with your elbows slightly bent. Exhale, stretching your arms straight out.

• Inhale again, bend your elbows slightly, and slowly drop your arms down until your thumbs touch the sides of your legs.

• Exhale one more time, then stand up straight.

**Daily Weigh-In:** _____ (weight in pounds)

**Workbook Assignment**: Write down how you felt after every meal and snack. Consider your hunger level, energy level, and overall mood. Rate how you were feeling from 1 to 5, with 1 being "dissatisfied" and 5 being "extremely satisfied."

| | | | | | |
|---|---|---|---|---|---|
| Breakfast | 1 | 2 | 3 | 4 | 5 |
| Snack | 1 | 2 | 3 | 4 | 5 |
| Lunch | 1 | 2 | 3 | 4 | 5 |
| Snack | 1 | 2 | 3 | 4 | 5 |
| Dinner | 1 | 2 | 3 | 4 | 5 |
| Evening Snack | 1 | 2 | 3 | 4 | 5 |

Visualize how your life will be different when you become fit on the Slim•Fast Plan. What do you have to look forward to?

_____

_____

_____

What particular things will keep you motivated to keep up your weight-loss efforts?

_____

_____

_____

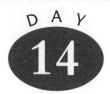

D A Y

14

> *Character is the ability to follow through on a project long after the mood has passed.*
>
> —Anonymous

Devise a daily affirmation that will help you stay your course on the weight-loss track for life. The next time you're feeling tempted to overindulge, repeat ten times, "I am healthy, I am strong. I am doing what's best for me."

## DAILY MENU

### BREAKFAST
1 Ultra Slim•Fast Meal On-The-Go Bar
4 ounces cranberry juice
Beverage, noncaloric

### MORNING SNACK
8 ounces nonfat fruit yogurt, artificially sweetened
Beverage, noncaloric

### LUNCH
1 Ultra Slim•Fast Cafe Mocha Powder Mix Shake
Beverage, noncaloric

**AFTERNOON SNACK**

**Vegetable Sticks**

    1 red pepper, washed, cored, seeded, and cut into strips

    1 stalk celery, washed and cut into strips

    1 tablespoon fat-free cream cheese

Beverage, noncaloric

**DINNER**

Garden Salad (page 110)

Split Pea Soup (page 110)

Herbed Whole-Grain Bread (page 111)

1/8 honeydew melon

Beverage, noncaloric

**EVENING SNACK**

1 Ultra Slim•Fast Nutritional Energy Snack Bar

Beverage, noncaloric

**DAY 14**   NUTRITIONAL INFORMATION

| Day Total | Calories | Protein | Carbohydrates | Fat | Fiber | Sodium | Cholesterol | Calcium |
|-----------|----------|---------|---------------|-----|-------|--------|-------------|---------|
|           | 1,422    | 70 g    | 248 g         | 21 g (13%) | 33 g | 1,174 mg | 30 mg | 1,375 mg |

# Garden Salad

*Total preparation time: 12 minutes*

1 small head red-leaf lettuce, outer leaves removed, washed, dried, and torn
   into bite-size pieces
1 small head romaine lettuce, outer leaves removed, washed, dried, and torn
   into bite-size pieces
1 large cucumber, peeled and thinly sliced
8 radishes, washed, trimmed, and thinly sliced
24 cherry tomatoes, washed and halved
1/2 cup fat-free dressing

In a large salad bowl, toss all ingredients except dressing. Dress immediately before serving.

SERVES 4

NUTRITIONAL INFORMATION PER SERVING

|  | Calories | Protein | Carbohydrates | Fat | Fiber | Sodium | Cholesterol | Calcium |
|---|---|---|---|---|---|---|---|---|
| **Garden Salad** | 74 | 3 g | 16 g | 1 g (10%) | 4 g | 37 mg | 0 mg | 56 mg |

# Split Pea Soup

*Total preparation time: 1 hour 10 minutes*

1 pound dried yellow or green split peas
2 teaspoons olive oil
3 cloves garlic, peeled and minced
5 cups chicken or vegetable stock
1 cup water

1.  Sort split peas to remove any debris. Rinse, drain, and set aside.
2.  Place olive oil in a 4- or 5-quart saucepan over medium-high heat. Add garlic and sauté until golden, 30 seconds. Add split peas, broth, and water, increase heat to high, and bring to a boil. Reduce heat to low, cover, and simmer until peas are tender when mashed, 45 minutes.

SERVES 4

NUTRITIONAL INFORMATION PER SERVING

|  | Calories | Protein | Carbohydrates | Fat | Fiber | Sodium | Cholesterol | Calcium |
|---|---|---|---|---|---|---|---|---|
| **Split Pea Soup** | 447 | 31 g | 73 g | 5 g (11%) | 16 g | 180 mg | 5 mg | 69 mg |

# Herbed Whole-Grain Bread

*Total preparation time: 5 minutes*

**4 teaspoons diet margarine**
**4 thick slices whole-grain bread**
**1/4 teaspoon garlic powder**
**1/2 teaspoon poppy seeds**
**1/2 teaspoon chives (or substitute your favorite herbs)**

1.  Preheat broiler.
2.  Spread a thin layer of margarine on bread and sprinkle with desired spices. Broil close to flame until edges are golden, 30 to 60 seconds.

SERVES 4

NUTRITIONAL INFORMATION PER SERVING

|  | Calories | Protein | Carbohydrates | Fat | Fiber | Sodium | Cholesterol | Calcium |
|---|---|---|---|---|---|---|---|---|
| **Herbed Whole-Grain Bread** | 94 | 3 g | 14 g | 3 g (29%) | 1 g | 187 mg | 0 mg | 37 mg |

**Exercise Must-Do:** Whether you choose to take a walk, strap on some in-line skates, or go for a bike ride, try exercising with a partner. You can be each other's personal trainer and motivate each other to push harder. Choose a friend, your spouse, or even your dog. No matter who you're with, you'll see that working out in tandem drives away boredom and makes exercise fun!

**Instant Stress Reliever:** To get into a relaxed state of being, apply some acupressure, which stimulates the same pressure points as acupuncture but uses fingers instead of needles. Find the "Third Eye," located between the eyebrows, in the indentation where the bridge of the nose meets the forehead. Breathe deeply and apply firm, steady pressure on each point for two to three minutes. The pressure should cause a mild aching sensation, but not pain.

**Daily Weigh-In:** _____ (weight in pounds)

**Workbook Assignment:** Write down how you felt after every meal and snack. Consider your hunger level, energy level, and overall mood. Rate how you were feeling from 1 to 5, with 1 being "dissatisfied" and 5 being "extremely satisfied."

| | | | | | |
|---|---|---|---|---|---|
| Breakfast | 1 | 2 | 3 | 4 | 5 |
| Snack | 1 | 2 | 3 | 4 | 5 |
| Lunch | 1 | 2 | 3 | 4 | 5 |
| Snack | 1 | 2 | 3 | 4 | 5 |
| Dinner | 1 | 2 | 3 | 4 | 5 |
| Evening Snack | 1 | 2 | 3 | 4 | 5 |

Visualize how your life will be different when you become fit on the Slim•Fast Plan. What do you have to look forward to?

_____

_____

_____

What particular things will keep you motivated to live the Slim•Fast Plan forever?

_____

_____

_____

# Your First Steps to Success

Congratulations: You've completed the 14-Day Plan. You've dedicated two weeks to your own fitness and health, and you've probably already begun to feel the results. Have you felt more relaxed? More energetic? Happier? Terrific. You've probably lost a few pounds—and even if it's only a start, at least you've seen that *you can do it*. You've seen that living healthy doesn't mean living a lifestyle of restrictions, deprivations, or denials.

So where do we go from here?

The following chapters discuss the basics of nutrition and exercise: why they're important for your health, and how you can work good health habits into your life—on your own terms. The 14-Day Plan gave you a sense of how great a new lifestyle can make you feel. But you can't stay on a prescribed plan forever. It's time to help you tailor a plan that fits comfortably into your life. It's time for you to create your own full-time Body•Mind•Life Makeover.

Say *yes* to life, *yes* to good health, and *yes* to yourself. Set yourself a new goal: to have the body and life you want. You'll only have yourself to thank.

# 5

# BALANCED NUTRITION FOR A HEALTHY LIFE®

Now that you've begun to learn just how great you can feel on the road to weight loss and fitness, it's time to give yourself the full treatment: the Body•Mind•Life Makeover.

Before you get started mapping out your new life plan, it's important to understand some basics about nutrition—the process that keeps your body working efficiently. In the past quarter-century, myths about nutrition have flown thick and fast through our culture, each one more alarming and irresistible than the last. We've been told we need to avoid all fat; that we should ban red meat from our diet; that we can indulge in as many cookies as we like—as long as they're fat-free. Wrong, wrong, wrong—and in this chapter you'll see why.

The truth is, trying to understand nutrition can be confusing, even discouraging—especially with the constant parade of new studies we're always hearing about in the news. Remember when researchers announced that margarine caused heart attacks in women? For a moment, many of us thought we could return to butter—until it turned out that butter was no better. Remember when oat bran, tofu, and green tea all made headlines? Ultimately, these foods all have their benefits, but none of them is the cancer or heart disease cure-all some might have believed. Fat became a nutritional villain, until it was suddenly dubbed an essential part of our diets. Pasta and bread—once nutritional darlings—are now the culprits behind such ills as obesity and diabetes. It's like the scene in the movie *Sleeper* where Woody Allen goes into the future, only to discover that organic rice been deemed unhealthy and that cigarette smoking can actually help you live longer.

Now here's a surprise: The basic definition of good nutrition hasn't really changed much in the past thirty years. It's still important to load up on fruits and vegetables, eat fat in moderation, and eat plenty of unrefined complex carbohydrates such as oatmeal, brown rice, and whole-grain bread. Consuming a variety of foods is still the best way to give your body a balanced supply of nutrients—better than throwing it all away in favor of whatever disease-fighter du jour was on the news last night. If you hear that your favorite vegetable can help prevent cancer, it's fine to include a few extra servings in your diet each week. What you shouldn't do is load up on that one veggie and forgo the rest.

Nutritional researchers know they'll never find one magic food that will keep our bodies healthy and prevent disease. That's why they recommend aiming for a rainbow diet that includes as many colors of fruits and vegetables as you can possibly get. The chemicals that put the purple in plums, the red in tomatoes, and the green in spinach—phytochemicals, as they're called—can help combat disease by neutralizing cancer-causing substances lurking within the body. Eating lots of produce will also help you get a wide variety of vitamins, including antioxidants that have been shown to help fight disease.

This is just one aspect of good nutrition. Another involves the kind of sensible advice your grandmother gave you: *Eat all foods in moderation.* The fact is, you don't need to banish any foods as long as you eat a nutritionally balanced diet. As you read on, you may be surprised to learn that you've been going overboard to avoid certain foods—and excited to find that making a small change in your diet can help improve your health and take off those stubborn pounds.

# The Truth About Fat

*Fat makes you fat; avoid it at all costs.* You've probably recited those words in your head time and time again. After all, high-fat foods *are* a concentrated source of calories, and when consumed in excess they can lead to obesity and raise your risk of heart disease and certain cancers. And carbohydrates and protein (which contain 4 calories per gram) have less than half the calories of fat (9 calories per gram).

So, isn't it better to avoid fat altogether? No, say experts. Just because a low-fat diet is good for you doesn't mean a no-fat diet is better. What's important is just to watch your fat intake, and not let it get away from you—something that's easy to do on the Slim•Fast Plan.

You should get no more than 30 percent of your total calories from fat, according to the U.S. Department of Agriculture's 1995 Dietary Guidelines for Americans. According to these guidelines, no more than 10 percent of your total calories should come from saturated fat, and no more than 10 percent from polyunsaturated fat. Since it was issued, though, nutrition experts have been debating the wisdom of this advice; many feel you should get only 20 to 25 percent of your calories from fat to maintain a healthy weight and help prevent cancer and heart disease. Others contend that if your diet is high in monounsaturated fats, you don't have to worry about going over the 30 percent mark. (A draft of the 2000 Dietary Guidelines, which were not finalized at press time, recommends a diet low in saturated fat and cholesterol and *moderate* in total fat.)

Following the Body•Mind•Life Makeover, you'll get about 20 percent of your total calories from fat, a low level that should help you lose weight and improve your health. At 1,400 to 1,500 calories per day (the weight-loss plan's allotment), you should be eating about 31 grams of fat each day. An Ultra Slim•Fast shake contains no more than 3 grams of fat, so the bulk of the fat in your diet will come from your meals and snacks. Although you should read labels for the fat content, you shouldn't make fat grams the sole determining factor in your diet. Simply choose foods that are naturally low in saturated fat and use olive, canola, and peanut oils, which are rich in monounsaturated fats.

Use the following chart as a guide to making wise food choices:

| Instead of . . . | Choose . . . |
|---|---|
| 2% milk<br>(1 cup: 121 cal, 5 g fat) | fat-free milk<br>(1 cup: 86 cal, 0.5 g fat) |
| corn oil<br>(1 tablespoon: 120 cal;<br>2 g saturated fat,<br>8 g polyunsaturated fat,<br>4 g monounsaturated fat) | olive oil<br>(1 tablespoon: 120 cal;<br>2 g saturated fat,<br>1 g polyunsaturated fat,<br>10 g monounsaturated fat) |
| dark meat chicken<br>(thigh, drumstick with skin)<br>(6 ounces: 430 cal, 27 g fat) | white meat chicken<br>(breast, skinless)<br>(6 ounces: 281 cal, 6 g fat) |
| cheddar cheese<br>(2 ounces: 229 cal, 19 g fat) | reduced-fat cheddar cheese<br>(2 ounces: 162 cal, 9 g fat) |
| prime rib steak<br>(6 ounces: 667 cal, 56 g fat) | beef top round<br>(6 ounces: 306 cal, 8 g fat) |
| croissant<br>(3 ounces: 345 cal, 18 g fat) | oat bran bagel<br>(3 ounces: 217 cal, 1 g fat) |
| doughnut<br>(2 ounces: 239 cal, 13 g fat) | graham crackers<br>(2 ounces: 243 cal, 6 g fat) |

## The Lowdown on Carbohydrates

In the early 1990s, we were in the midst of a love affair with carbohydrates. Pasta, bread, and fat-free cookies were seen as freebies: Since they had little fat, many thought they'd be a great way to help lose weight. We let portions go to the wind—and we watched ourselves get fatter, not thinner. The failure of these high-carb diets caused the pendulum to swing the other way. Suddenly carbohydrates were the culprits behind every health ill from diabetes to heart disease to obesity. Now high-protein diets are the latest fad, as we struggle to divorce ourselves from starchy foods.

Like any food hailed as a panacea, carbohydrates have toppled off their high pedestal. After all, they do contain calories, and enough of those calories can make you fat. That said, the carbohydrate equation becomes a bit more complicated. A huge variety of foods fall into the carb category: fruits, vegetables, and sugar are the simple carbs, and pasta, bread, potatoes, and other starches are complex carbs. Simple or complex, your body breaks down all the carbohydrates into a single sugar called glucose, which is used for fuel. That's about where the similarities between the different types of carbs end.

Nutritionally, all carbohydrates are not created equal. A high-fiber, low-sugar carb (a peach, for instance) is a lot less calorie-dense than a low-fiber, high-sugar carb (a piece of peach pie). Your body breaks down low-fiber, highly processed carbs much faster, which is why you get a quick energy boost after eating sweetened cereal or a glass of juice. Your body breaks down unrefined, high-fiber carbs (fresh fruits and vegetables, whole-grain bread and rice, slow-cooked oatmeal) more gradually, which gives you a steadier stream of energy and helps you feel sated.

By far, the carb we eat the most of is refined sugar, usually in the context of cookies, cakes, and other snack foods. As most of us now regularly buy fat-free and reduced-fat treats, we have traded in fat for sugar. The average American woman has added 27 pounds of sugar, corn syrup, and other high-calorie sweeteners to her annual intake since 1986—around the same time reduced-fat products appeared in the supermarket. After all, food manufacturers knew that you wouldn't buy a product that didn't taste good, so they loaded those yummy fat-free brownie bars and coffee cakes with extra sugar. That way, you wouldn't miss the fat.

Unfortunately, extra sugar means extra calories. In fact, many reduced-fat and fat-free products contain nearly as many calories as their full-fat counterparts. Just compare the label of reduced-fat peanut butter with that of its original counterpart. A 2-tablespoon serving of the reduced-fat version contains 180 calories, 12 grams of fat, and 5 grams of sugar. The regular version contains 190 calories, 16 grams of fat, and 2 grams of sugar. (The 10-calorie savings gets you more than twice the amount of sugar, and gives you less of the heart-healthy monounsaturated fat found in peanut butter.) You'll probably find that reduced-fat cookies are no calorie bargains either. Of course, it's fine to replace your regular cookies or ice cream with reduced-fat versions—just don't give yourself license to eat *more*. Stick with the serving-size portion, and remember that if you go overboard you can easily eat *far* more calories than you normally would.

Keep in mind, too, that *sugar is not a bad food* that deserves to be banned from your diet. Foods with a lot of refined sugar, however, usually contain little nutrition and a lot of calories. Your best bet is to save the sugary sweets for special occasions. On the other hand, the little sugar packet on the table that you use to flavor your coffee won't destroy your diet. If you prefer sugar to saccharine or aspartame, allow yourself a little of the real thing. It has only 16 calories per teaspoon. Just use it sparingly.

The carbs that give you the biggest nutritional bang for your buck are those that are high in fiber, an indigestible form of carbohydrate found only in plants. Eating fiber-rich foods can make you feel fuller for longer, lower your cholesterol, and provide the bulk necessary to promote regularity and prevent constipation. What's more, the higher the dietary fiber in a food, the less fat and calories it contains, and the more slowly it's absorbed by the body.

Since fiber slows digestion, you feel fuller between meals—which can actually help you eat less at the next meal. A study from the International Life Sciences Institute found that eating high-fiber foods for breakfast or lunch appears to reduce food intake at the next meal. At up to 5 grams per serving, Slim•Fast shakes are a good source of fiber. Here are some other high-fiber stars, any of which you can include in your personal eating plan:

| Food | Serving Size | Moderate Fiber (2 to 4 g) | High Fiber (5+ g) |
|------|------------|---------------------------|-------------------|
| Breads | 1 slice/muffin | whole wheat, cracked wheat, bran muffin | |
| | 4 crackers | rye wafers | |
| Cereals | 1 ounce | Bran Flakes, Raisin Bran, Shredded Wheat, oatmeal, Corn Bran | All Bran, Multi-Bran Chex |
| Vegetables | 1/2 cup | beets, broccoli, brussels sprouts, cabbage, carrots, corn, green beans, green peas, frozen spinach (boiled) | |
| | 1 medium | baked potato with skin | corn on the cob |
| Fruits | 1 medium | apple with peel, date, fig, mango, nectarine, orange, pear, banana | |
| | 1/2 cup | applesauce (unsweetened), raspberries, blackberries | cooked prunes |
| Legumes | 1/2 cup | baked beans, black beans, garbanzos, kidney or pinto beans, lentils, lima beans | |

# How Much Protein Do You Really Need?

High-protein diets have surged in popularity, billing themselves as the final answer to the obesity question. Since we've gotten fat on carbohydrates and high-fat foods, we should be able to lose weight using a protein-rich diet. The truth is, you can lose weight on a high-protein diet the same as you can on any other diet. The real trouble is that these diets don't have much staying power. After a while, we get sick of eating meat, chicken, and fish for breakfast, lunch, and dinner. And we begin to crave the bread that's missing from our sandwiches and the popcorn and pretzels that are banned as snacks.

What's more, many nutritionists frown on high-protein diets because they don't provide you with the balanced nutrition your body needs. The Body•Mind•Life Makeover will give you the *proper* balance of protein, carbs, and fat—based on the sensible guidelines of the U.S. Department of Agriculture. On the Makeover, you'll be getting about 20 percent of your calories from fat, 55 percent from carbohydrates, and 25 percent from protein. The Slim•Fast eating plan calls for you to consume about 88 grams of protein a day. Two Slim•Fast shakes plus one 6-ounce serving of meat, chicken, fish, or vegetable protein should fulfill your protein requirement.

Protein is an essential nutrient that is the basis of all life; after water, it's the most plentiful substance in the human body, composing most of your muscle mass, skin, hair, eyes, and nails. And the real secret to having sustained energy throughout the day lies in eating the right combination of protein and carbohydrates—which you'll find on the Slim•Fast Makeover. Carbs will cause an immediate rise in your blood sugar; protein will boost it later; and your energy levels will be sustained until your next meal. The goal to shoot for is ½ gram of high-quality protein for every pound of your goal body weight.

What's high-quality protein? Just as with carbohydrates and fats, the key to protein lies in choosing the right kinds. Two of our most popular protein choices, red meat and dairy products, have traditionally contained large amounts of saturated fats and cholesterol. But advances in biotechnology have brought lower-fat options. Beef has slimmed down, and some cuts—like beef top round (select) and eye of round (select)—are leaner than some cuts of chicken. Skim milk is, of course, virtually fat-free. If you don't care for the taste, there are even new brands of skim milk that claim to taste just like whole milk. You can also choose fat-free and reduced-fat cheese, yogurt, sour cream, and egg products. All of these are packed with protein with little or no saturated fat or cholesterol.

Protein from plant sources packs an even larger nutritional punch. In the average American's diet, plant sources—grains, vegetables, legumes, soy, nuts, and seeds—account for only one-third of the amount of protein consumed, even though they contain virtually no fat and are loaded with phytochemicals that can help ward off disease. By replacing some of your animal protein consumption with plant proteins, you'll be doing yourself a favor. Some rich plant-protein foods include: ½ cup cooked soybeans (11 grams of protein), 4 ounces firm tofu (9 g), ½ cup kidney beans (9 g), 1 cup cooked bulgur (6 g), 1 cup cooked spaghetti (7 g), or 1 cup cooked oatmeal (6 g).

# Calcium: Are You Getting Enough?

A whopping 80 percent of women don't get enough calcium, which is thought to help protect against osteoporosis later in life. This is because many calcium-rich foods like cheese and ice cream also tend to be high in fat and calories. So if you're trying to lose weight, you're probably also trying to avoid these foods.

Long hailed as the best bone-builder around, calcium has an amazing host of other health benefits. In a recent study from the National Heart, Lung, and Blood Institute, researchers tested the effects of three eating plans to see which one was most effective at preventing hypertension: standard American fare (high in animal protein and refined carbohydrates) was compared against a diet high in fruits and vegetables and a combination diet that was rich in fruits, vegetables, and low-fat dairy products (similar to the Slim•Fast eating plan). The study found that the combination diet was as effective at controlling high blood pressure as some antihypertensive medications, while the diet without the low-fat dairy allotment was only about half as effective. Calcium is believed to reduce blood pressure by causing the production of a chemical that causes blood vessels to relax and open up.

Other research suggests that a diet rich in calcium may help ease premenstrual syndrome. In one study from Columbia-Presbyterian Medical Center in New York, thirty-three women took 1,000 mg of calcium carbonate supplements for three months and then took a placebo for three additional months. The women reported a 50 percent reduction in premenstrual symptoms (bloating, breast tenderness, irritability) and menstrual symptoms (back pain, cramping) when they were taking the calcium, and 78 percent reported feeling better overall while taking calcium compared to the placebo.

Scientific evidence also finds that high-calcium foods pack more punch than supplements. You should get 1,000 mg of calcium daily; here's a list of ten top calcium-rich foods:

| Food | Serving | Calcium (mg) | Calories | Fat (grams) |
|---|---|---|---|---|
| Fat-free (skim) milk | 1 cup | 301 | 86 | Less than 1 |
| Yogurt, plain, nonfat | 1 cup | 487 | 137 | Less than 1 |
| Ultra Slim•Fast Ready-to-Drink milk-based shake | 11-ounce can | 400 | 220 | 3 |
| Tofu (processed with calcium sulfate) | 4 ounces | 397 | 86 | 5 |
| Calcium-fortified orange juice | 8 ounces | 350 | 110 | 0 |
| Salmon, canned, drained with bones | 3 ounces | 203 | 130 | 6 |
| Orange | 1 medium | 52 | 62 | 0 |
| Broccoli, boiled, drained | 1/2 cup | 36 | 22 | Less than 1 |
| Romaine lettuce | 2 cups, chopped | 40 | 16 | 0 |
| Cottage cheese, 1% milkfat | 4 ounces | 99 | 79 | 1 |

# The Key Vitamins and Minerals You Need

Vitamins and minerals are key nutrients your body uses to help the normal functioning of cells. They can help promote good vision, form normal blood cells, create strong bones and teeth, and ensure the proper functioning of the heart and brain. There are thirteen vitamins we need most: vitamins A, C, D, E, K, and eight B-complex vitamins—thiamine, riboflavin, niacin, $B_6$, pantothenic acid, biotin, folic acid, and $B_{12}$. Each of these vitamins carries out specific functions, and if a certain vitamin isn't supplied through our diet over a long period of time, a particular deficiency disease usually results.

Like vitamins, minerals are also essential for your body to perform a host of vital functions, from basic bone formation to the regulation of your heartbeat to the normal functioning of digestion. Although there are sixty different types of minerals in your body, only twenty-two essential minerals are necessary for your diet. These include large or macro-minerals, including calcium, magnesium, phosphorus, potassium, and sodium, and small or micro-minerals such as chromium, copper, iron, manganese, molybdenum, selenium, and zinc.

Since vitamins and minerals can ward off certain diseases caused by deficiencies, you might assume that the more, the better. But science says otherwise. The bulk of the vitamin research studies indicate that vitamins and minerals don't bestow additional health benefits if taken in amounts much greater than the U.S. government's recommended DV (Daily Value). In fact, some vitamins (like vitamins A and D) can be toxic if taken in excessive amounts.

Unless your doctor advises you to take a certain supplement, you can meet your vitamin and mineral needs by drinking two Slim•Fast shakes a day—which are fortified with up to twenty-four essential vitamins and minerals—along with a variety of fruits and vegetables and a balanced meal. Each milk-based shake gives you more than a third of the DV for most vitamins and minerals, including calcium, vitamin E, and vitamin C. You should have no trouble getting the rest of the vitamins and minerals you need from the foods you eat. The two charts on pages 126–129 contain a quick rundown of the essential vitamins and minerals—which foods to get them from and how your body uses them.

# Vitamins: Where to Get Them, How You Use Them

| Vitamin | Food Source | What It Does |
|---|---|---|
| Vitamin A | Liver, eggs, fortified milk, carrots, tomatoes, apricots, cantaloupe, fish | Promotes good vision, helps form and maintain healthy skin and mucous membranes; may protect against some cancers |
| Vitamin C | Citrus fruits, strawberries, tomatoes | Promotes healthy gums, capillaries, and teeth; aids iron absorption; may block production of nitrosamines; maintains normal connective tissue; aids in healing wounds |
| Vitamin D | Fortified milk, fish; also produced by the body in response to sunlight | Promotes strong bones and teeth; necessary for absorption of calcium |
| Vitamin E | Nuts, vegetable oils, whole grains, olives, asparagus, spinach | Protects tissue against damage from cancer-causing substances; important in formation of red blood cells; helps body use vitamin K. May prevent or alleviate coronary heart disease. |
| Vitamin K | Body produces about half of daily needs; cauliflower, broccoli, cabbage, spinach, cereals, soybeans, beef liver | Aids in clotting of blood |
| Vitamin $B_1$ (thiamine) | Whole grains, dried beans, lean meats (especially pork), fish | Helps release energy from carbohydrates; necessary for healthy brain and nerve cells and for functioning of heart |
| Vitamin $B_2$ (riboflavin) | Nuts, dairy products, liver | Aids in release of energy from foods; interacts with other B vitamins |

| Vitamin | Food Source | What It Does |
| --- | --- | --- |
| Vitamin $B_3$ (niacin) | Nuts, dairy products, liver | Aids in release of energy from foods; involved in synthesis of DNA; maintains normal functioning of skin, nerves, and digestive system |
| Vitamin $B_5$ (pantothenic acid) | Whole grains, dried beans, eggs, nuts | Aids in the release of energy from foods; essential for synthesis of numerous body materials |
| Vitamin $B_6$ (pyridoxine) | Whole grains, dried beans, eggs, nuts | Important in chemical reactions of proteins and amino acids; involved in normal functioning of brain and formation of red blood cells |
| Vitamin $B_{12}$ | Liver, beef, eggs, milk, shellfish | Necessary for development of red blood cells; maintains normal functioning of nervous system |
| Folic acid | Liver, wheat bran, leafy green vegetables, beans, grains | Important in synthesis of DNA; acts together with $B_{12}$ in the production of hemoglobin (which carries oxygen through the blood) |
| Biotin | Yeast, eggs, liver, milk | Important in formation of fatty acids; helps metabolize amino acids and carbohydrates |

Source: University of California, Berkeley, *The Wellness Encyclopedia* (Houghton Mifflin, 1991).

# Minerals: Where to Get Them, How You Use Them

| Mineral | Food Source | What It Does |
|---|---|---|
| Calcium | Milk and milk products, sardines and salmon eaten with bone, dark green leafy vegetables, shellfish, hard water | Builds bones and teeth, maintains bone density and strength; helps prevent osteoporosis; helps regulate heartbeat, blood clotting, muscle contraction, and nerve conduction |
| Chloride | Table salt, fish | Maintains normal fluid shifts; balances blood pH; forms stomach acid to aid in digestion |
| Magnesium | Wheat bran, whole grains, raw leafy green vegetables, nuts (especially almonds and cashews), soybeans, bananas, apricots, spices | Aids in bone growth; aids function of nerves and muscle, including regulation of normal heart rhythm |
| Phosphorus | Meats, poultry, fish, cheese, egg yolks, dried peas and beans, milk and milk products, soft drinks, nuts; present in almost all foods | Aids in bone growth and strengthening of teeth; important in energy metabolism |
| Potassium | Oranges and orange juice, bananas, dried fruits, peanut butter, dried peas and beans, potatoes, coffee, tea, cocoa, yogurt, molasses, meat | Promotes regular heartbeat; active in muscle contraction; regulates transfer of nutrients to cells; controls water balance in body tissues and cells; helps regulate blood pressure |
| Sodium | Table salt, salt added to prepared foods, baking soda | Helps regulate water balance in body; plays a role in maintaining blood pressure |
| Chromium | Meat, cheese, whole grains, dried peas and beans, peanuts | Important for glucose metabolism; may be a cofactor for insulin |

| Mineral | Food Source | What It Does |
|---|---|---|
| Copper | Shellfish, nuts, beef and pork liver, cocoa powder, chocolate, kidneys, dried beans, raisins, corn oil margarine | Formation of red blood cells; cofactor in absorbing iron into blood cells; helps produce several respiratory enzymes |
| Fluorine (fluoride) | Fluoridated water and foods grown or cooked in it; fish, tea, gelatin | Contributes to solid bone and tooth formation; may help prevent osteoporosis |
| Iodine | Primarily from iodized salt, but also seafood, seaweed food products, vegetables grown in iodine-rich areas, vegetable oil | Necessary for normal function of the thyroid gland and for normal cell function; keeps skin, hair, and nails healthy; prevents goiter |
| Iron | Liver, kidneys, red meats, egg yolks, peas, beans, nuts, dried fruits, green leafy vegetables, enriched grain products | Essential to formation of hemoglobin (which carries oxygen through the blood); part of several enzymes and proteins in the body |
| Manganese | Nuts, whole grains, vegetables, fruits, instant coffee, tea, cocoa powder, beets, egg yolks | Required for normal bone growth and development, normal reproduction, and cell function |
| Molybdenum | Peas, beans, cereal grains, organ meats, some dark green vegetables | Important for normal cell function |
| Selenium | Fish, shellfish, red meat, egg yolks, chicken, garlic, tuna, tomatoes | Complements vitamin E to fight cell damage by certain cancer-causing substances called free radicals |
| Zinc | Oysters, crabmeat, beef, liver, eggs, poultry, brewer's yeast, whole wheat bread | Maintains taste and smell acuity; normal growth and sexual development; important for fetal growth and wound healing |

Source: University of California, Berkeley, *The Wellness Encyclopedia* (Houghton Mifflin, 1991).

# Water: The Forgotten Nutrient

You've heard it a thousand times before: Drink eight glasses of water a day to stay healthy. A vital nutrient that makes up 55 to 60 percent of your body weight, water stabilizes body temperature, carries nutrients to and waste away from cells, and is needed for cells to function. Water also aids in digestion and helps prevent constipation, and it works wonders at filling you up when you drink it with a meal.

Now, let's be honest. Do you actually make a concerted effort to drink eight 8-ounce glasses of fluid each day, plus another three or four after you've been out in the heat or exercising? Or, like most of us, do you just take a drink when you feel thirsty?

Unfortunately, judging by your own feeling of thirst may not be enough: Often we don't feel thirsty until our bodies reach a dehydration danger point. You may lose up to two quarts of water (4 pounds) before thirst prompts you to start drinking. In general, feeling thirsty means dehydration is setting in.

Not drinking enough water can be damaging to your health. Getting dehydrated during a workout can lead to premature fatigue and raises your risk of heat exhaustion and heatstroke on a hot day. Dehydration can cause fatigue and make you feel headachy, dizzy, and nauseated. And not drinking enough water on a day-to-day basis can leave you feeling out of sorts. Case in point: People who drink three or fewer glasses of water or other fluids a day were more likely to suffer symptoms from morning grogginess to dry skin, according to a recent survey of three thousand people conducted by the Nutrition Information Center at the New York Hospital–Cornell Medical Center in New York.

The survey also found that although most people consume an average of 8.5 cups a day of hydrating beverages—milk, juice, caffeine-free soft drinks, and water—they also drink an average of 4.5 cups of dehydrating beverages—coffee, tea, caffeinated soft drinks, and alcohol. Alcohol and caffeine are diuretics, substances that cause the body to lose water through urination.

Fortunately, you shouldn't have much difficulty getting the water you need if you follow these basic rules of thumb:

● **Get the equivalent of 8 glasses of water a day.** If you drink coffee, alcohol, or other dehydrating beverages, offset the loss of water by drinking an additional glass of water for every dehydrating beverage you drink. This means 10 cups of water a day if you have a cup of java in the morning and a diet cola with lunch.

● **Drink before you exercise, as well as during and afterward.** Ideally, you should drink two 8-ounce cups of water two hours before your activity. You'll lose any excess through urination before you begin to exercise. If you can't drink water two hours in advance, have an 8-ounce glass just before you begin. While you're exercising, drink 6 to 12 ounces of water every fifteen to twenty minutes, especially when you're outdoors in the heat.

● **Use your weight as a guide.** Weigh yourself before and after your workout—preferably unclothed, since sweaty clothes weigh more than dry ones. For each pound less that you weigh after your workout, drink a pint (two cups) of water to replace the water you lost as sweat. Keep in mind that you lose about one pound of water for every 300 calories you burn.

● **Keep a pitcher of water nearby.** Place it on your desk at work or on the kitchen table. You'll be reminded to drink throughout the day, and you may find it helps control your hunger. What you think is hunger may really be a craving for water.

## Foods That Prevent Disease

Even in this technological day and age, scientists would be hard pressed to create the perfect food—a food that contains all the nutrients that your body needs. Slim•Fast and other meal replacement products contain nutrients such as fat, protein, and carbohydrates as well as fiber and a host of essential vitamins and minerals. But they don't contain the hundreds of other hidden nutrients that scientists continue to learn more about every day. These are tiny molecules called phytochemicals that act almost like medicine to impart health benefits beyond basic nutrition. For instance, lycopene (a phytochemical that gives tomatoes their red color) made all the headlines when researchers from Harvard University and the Dana Farber Cancer Institute discovered that it may reduce the risk of prostate cancer.

Some phytochemicals reduce your risk of cancer or heart disease; others prevent gastrointestinal problems. All can help you stay healthy, and you won't find most of them in a pill. The fact is, scientists still don't know how all the phytochemicals work, whether they would be more effective in megadoses, and whether taking them in combination might increase (or counteract) their effects. For instance, lycopene might work hand in hand with antioxidant vitamins in fruits and vegetables to bolster cancer-preventive effects.

How can you get a dose of this medicine? Eat a variety of fruits and vegetables to get a variety of phytochemicals. Here are just a few of the key phytochemicals you need:

## Examples of Foods That Can Prevent Disease

| Type of Phytochemical | Source | Potential Benefit |
| --- | --- | --- |
| Antiadhesion component (not fully identified) | Cranberry juice cocktail | May improve urinary tract health |
| Carotenoids | | |
|     Alpha-carotene | Carrots | Neutralize free radicals that may cause damage to cells, turning a normal cell into a cancerous one |
|     Beta-carotene | Fruits, vegetables | |
|     Lutein | Green vegetables | |
|     Lycopene | Tomato products (ketchup, sauces, etc.) | |
|     Zeaxanthin | Eggs, citrus, corn | |
| Dietary Fiber | | |
|     Insoluble fiber | Wheat bran, vegetables | May reduce risk of breast or colon cancer |
|     Soluble fiber | Oats, barley, fruits | Reduce risk of cardiovascular disease (CVD) |

| Type of Phytochemical | Source | Potential Benefit |
|---|---|---|
| Flavonoids | | |
|     Anthocyanidins | Fruits | Neutralize free radicals, |
|     Catechins | Tea | may reduce risk of cancer |
|     Flavanones | Citrus | |
|     Flavones | Fruits/vegetables | |
| Glucosinolates, indoles, isothiocyanates sulphoraphane | Cruciferous vegetables (broccoli, kale, horseradish) | Neutralize free radicals, stimulate anti-cancer enzymes |
| Phenols | | |
|     Caffeic acid | Fruits, vegetables, | Antioxidant-like activities may |
|     Ferulic acid | citrus | reduce risk of degenerative diseases, heart disease, eye disease |
| Phytoestrogens | | |
|     Isoflavones | | |
|         Diadzein | Soybeans and | May protect against heart disease |
|         Genistein | soy-based foods | and some cancers; may lower LDL cholesterol |
|     Lignans | Flax, rye, vegetables | |
| Prebiotics/probiotics | | |
|     Lactobacillus | Yogurt, Jerusalem artichokes, shallots, onion powder | May improve quality of intestinal microflora |
|     Fructo-oligosaccharides | | |
| Saponins | Soybeans, soy foods, protein-containing foods | May lower LDL cholesterol; contains anti-cancer enzymes |
| Sulfides/Thiols | | |
|     Diallyl sulfide | Onion, garlic, olives, | Lower LDL cholesterol, maintain |
|     Allyl methyl trisulfide | leeks, scallions, | healthy immune system |
|     Dithoilthiones | cruciferous vegetables | |

Source: International Food Information Council

# Living a Vegetarian Lifestyle

Like millions of Americans, you may have chosen to lead a vegetarian lifestyle. Most people who have made such food choices will find that a vegetarian lifestyle fits perfectly with the Body•Mind•Life Makeover.* Vegetarian diets tend to be rich in fiber, complex carbohydrates, and many vitamins and minerals, including the antioxidants vitamin C and beta-carotene. Although you may eat less protein than a nonvegetarian, chances are you're getting enough to meet the protein DV. Some vegetarians may be at risk for deficiencies in iron, calcium, copper, zinc, manganese, or vitamin $B_{12}$. Fortunately, the Slim•Fast products are all fortified with these vitamins and minerals as well as protein. Using two Slim•Fast meal replacements a day and a carefully planned sensible meal should ensure that you have adequate amounts of the nutrients you need. The following foods are good sources for bolstering your intake of nutrients usually from animal proteins:

- Protein: Lentils, tofu, nuts, seeds, tempeh, peas
- Iron: Dried beans, spinach, chard, blackstrap molasses, bulgur, dried fruit
- Calcium: Collard greens, broccoli, kale, turnip greens, fortified soy milk or fruit juices, fortified tofu

* Slim•Fast products contain milk protein, so strict vegan dieters should take note.

Now that you've got the nutritional basics under your belt, you're ready to move on to designing your own personal makeover. It's time to transform your body and mind to get the life you've always wanted. This next chapter will give you the road map, but ultimately you're the one behind the wheel. Bon voyage!

# 6

# DESIGNING YOUR OWN PERSONAL MAKEOVER

I t's time to ask yourself: Am I ready to take charge of my life? Am I ready to become the master of my weight, my body, and my future?

Whether or not you're aware of it, you've already taken the reins. The 14-Day Plan showed you how it's done; you've learned the basics of nutrition and why the plan works. Now it's time to do it yourself.

When you give yourself the Body•Mind•Life Makeover, you'll be doing just that. *You* will choose the foods you eat, the exercises you do, and the ways you manage stress. You will map out a personal makeover that fits into your own unique lifestyle.

Of course, you have to follow a basic framework. (You can't expect to lose weight if you exercise only five minutes a day or eat a huge slice of cheesecake for dessert every night!) The next two chapters give you the rules of the Body•Mind•Life Makeover, and show you how to get started.

Although there are rules to follow, you'll have a lot of flexibility in the options you choose—from what you eat to how you exercise to what kinds of relaxation techniques are best for you. Having the freedom to personalize your own Body•Mind•Life Makeover will make it easier to stay on the plan for good. It's a plan you'll be happy to live with; you won't even *want* to drop it once you reach your goal.

If you've ever seen a cosmetic makeover on a TV talk show, you must have wondered what happened after the cameras were turned off and the subject went home to try to re-create her new look. After all, she had a professional stylist to cut and blow-dry her hair, a makeup artist to play up her face's best features, and a personal shopper to pick out an outfit that flattered her body type. Since the show obviously couldn't pay to monitor her look year-round, you can bet she went back to looking like her old self once she washed her hair, reapplied her makeup, and donned an outfit from her own closet.

The trouble with many beauty makeovers is that stylists don't teach the subject the skills she needs to transform herself day after day. And they usually don't think to do a makeover that can be easily replicated under a time crunch and tight budget.

Allowing you to design a plan that fits into your life and giving you the tools to follow through with it—these are exactly the goals of the Body•Mind•Life Makeover. Rather than seeing the results of your makeover in the blink of an eye—and watching them fade just as fast—you'll see a steady transformation. You'll gradually take off weight and see a sculpted body begin to emerge. You'll notice that you have a little more energy each day, and find that you actually start to *crave* physical activity. You'll begin to have more confidence in yourself until you feel like you can accomplish anything. You'll have an increasing sense of well-being. Then, one day, you'll realize you finally have the life you were looking for.

Margaret Mathis from Huntsville, Alabama, can't believe how much the Slim•Fast Plan has changed her body and her perspective on life:

> When I was fat, I was depressed and miserable. I didn't want people taking pictures of me, and I didn't like going to the store. I would take my child with me so people would know that I just had a baby. I was kind of quiet and stand-offish.
>
> When I started Slim•Fast, I went from a size 14 to a size 2. I was shocked and excited because I didn't think I could do it. All the vitamins and minerals in the shake boosted my energy and helped me keep going—to keep running after my one-year-old daughter. Now my whole perspective on life has changed, and I'm no longer intimidated by anybody. I feel like I can go anywhere and talk to anybody. My arms, legs, and waist are slim. This beautiful body was waiting to come out, and I had no idea until I started Slim•Fast.

# How to Design Your Personal Makeover

You'll be designing three distinct plans that should fit easily into your daily lifestyle: an eating plan, an exercise plan, and a relaxation plan. In this chapter, you'll be designing your eating plan. In the next chapter, you'll be designing a plan for exercise and relaxation, which work hand in hand to reduce stress, boost energy, and help you feel great about your body and your life. The key to making the Body•Mind•Life Makeover work for you is choosing the recipes and lifestyle activities you enjoy most; that's what the Body•Mind•Life Makeover is all about—finding your own way.

Once you've begun creating your personal plan, you'll need to keep track of your progress. At the end of this book, you'll find a Personal Makeover Diary you can use to track the first four weeks of your new plan. Each day you should write down everything you've eaten, along with your estimated total calorie count. You should also make note of the exercise you did (and your estimated calorie burn) and the relaxation techniques you used. You should also record your daily weight, and make general notes—on recipes you liked, whether a particular workout felt great or seemed too strenuous, and so on. *Keeping the daily workout diary is a vital part of this plan.* It allows you to see what works and what doesn't. It also lets you know whether you've suffered a lapse here or there by not getting enough exercise or by overindulging in sweet desserts. After you've finished your first month, you should continue with your diary; buy a notebook and keep it nearby, or even just photocopy the blank pages at the back of this book before you begin.

# Creating Your Personal Eating Plan

After following the 14-Day Plan, you're probably in one of two places: Either you've lost weight and want to lose some more, or you've lost weight and want to maintain the loss. Most likely, you fall into the first category—which means you'll be creating a weight-loss eating plan. At some point (whether you're there now or later), you'll reach your goal weight—at which point you can design a weight-maintenance plan to help keep it off for life.

## WEIGHT-LOSS EATING PLAN

To lose weight, you'll be on a 1,400- to 1,500-calorie-a-day plan that gives you two Slim•Fast shakes or Meal On-The-Go Bars instead of two regular meals, just as you had on the 14-Day Plan. Your goal should be to lose 1 to 2 pounds per week. (Some dieters may need to eat slightly more or less than what is on the plan to achieve this slow but steady weight loss; see below for details.)

And here's where the variety kicks in: For your third meal, you can choose from among the dozens of breakfast, lunch, and dinner recipes in this chapter. For instance, if you decide to have a shake for breakfast and another for lunch, you can choose a dinner recipe. If the next day you decide to have a shake for breakfast and dinner, you can whip up one of the quick and delicious lunch recipes. To control hunger between meals, you should also have two or three daily snacks between meals. Choose a Slim•Fast nutritional snack bar, or a snack from the list on the following pages.

---

*Remember, for weight loss it's:*

## Shake • Shake • Meal

**BREAKFAST:** Slim•Fast Shake or Meal On-The-Go Bar

**SNACK:** 1 piece of fruit, 1 cup raw vegetables, or a 60- to 90-calorie snack

**LUNCH:** Slim•Fast Shake or Meal On-The-Go Bar

**SNACK:** 1 piece of fruit, 1 cup raw vegetables, or a 60- to 90-calorie snack

**SNACK:** Slim•Fast Snack Bar or a 100- to 150-calorie snack

**DINNER:** Large tossed salad; 6 ounces of protein (meat, chicken, fish, or soy/vegetable protein); 3 servings of cooked vegetables; 1 serving starch (1/2 baked potato, 1 small ear of corn, or 1/2 cup rice/pasta); 1 piece of fruit for dessert

**BEVERAGES:** Drink 8 glasses of water or other caffeine-free, noncaloric beverages each day, and an extra for every caffeinated beverage you also consume

If you are small-framed or have been advised by your doctor to consume fewer calories per day, you can adjust the plan from 1,400 calories a day to 1,200. Reduce entrée size to 4 ounces of lean meat, fish, poultry, or vegetable protein at dinner; have two snacks daily instead of three.

Note: You should be losing about 1 to 2 pounds per week, the healthiest way to lose weight. If you are losing more than that, you should eat more to slow the rate of weight loss. Start by adding one extra snack a day and adding an extra serving of starch with your meal. Continue to increase by this amount until your weight loss slows to 1 to 2 pounds per week.

# Weight–Maintenance Eating Plan

To maintain your weight after you've reached your goal, you should be consuming about 300 to 500 calories more than you were consuming on the

---

*For weight maintenance, it's:*

## Meal • Shake • Meal

**BREAKFAST:** 1 1/2 cups high-fiber cereal, 1 cup fat-free milk, 1 piece fruit *or* 1 Slim•Fast Shake or Meal On-The-Go Bar

**SNACK:** 1 piece of fruit, 1 cup raw vegetables, or a 60- to 90-calorie snack

**LUNCH:** 1 sandwich (2 ounces luncheon meat or cheese, 3 tomato slices, 2 lettuce leaves, 1/2 cup shredded carrots, 2 slices bread); 1 cup artificially sweetened nonfat yogurt or 1 piece of fruit or 1 Slim•Fast Shake or Meal On-The-Go Bar

**SNACK:** 1 piece of fruit, 1 cup raw vegetables, or a 60- to 90-calorie snack

**SNACK:** 1 Slim•Fast Snack Bar or a 100- to 150-calorie snack

**DINNER:** Vegetable soup or side salad; 6 ounces of protein (meat, chicken, fish, or soy/vegetable protein); 3 servings of steamed or grilled vegetables; 1 serving of starch (potato, rice, pasta, etc.); 1 piece of fruit for dessert

**BEVERAGES:** Drink 8 glasses of water or other caffeine-free, noncaloric beverage each day, and one extra for every caffeinated beverage you also consume.

weight-loss plan. On the flip side, you should be consuming about 300 to 500 calories *less* than you were eating before you lost the weight. The easiest way to do this is to replace one Slim•Fast shake or Meal On-The-Go Bar with a second sensible meal. You'll continue to have one shake or meal bar each day for breakfast, lunch, or dinner, and then eat sensibly the rest of the day. You should also continue to have two or three daily snacks between meals.

# Slim•Fast Shakes and Bars— The Cornerstone of the Plan

Here's a list of Slim•Fast products you can use to replace meals or snacks. The shakes and Meal On-The-Go Bars can be used in place of a breakfast, lunch, or dinner; the nutritional snack bars help fill in between meals.

## Ready-to-Drink Shakes

**MILK-BASED**

Cappuccino Delight
Rich Chocolate Royale
French Vanilla

Strawberries 'n Cream
Creamy Milk Chocolate
Dark Chocolate Fudge

**SOY-AND-MILK-BASED**

Orange-Strawberry-Banana
Apple-Cranberry-Raspberry
Orange-Pineapple

# Slim•Fast Powders

**ULTRA SLIM•FAST (UP TO 5 GRAMS FIBER PER SERVING)**

Chocolate Royale          Chocolate Malt
French Vanilla            Chocolate Fudge
Strawberry Supreme        Juice Mixable
Café Mocha                Milk Chocolate

**SLIM•FAST (2 GRAMS FIBER PER SERVING)**

Chocolate                 Vanilla
Chocolate Malt            Strawberry

# Ultra Slim•Fast Nutritional Snack Bars

Peanut Butter Crunch
Rich Chewy Caramel
Crispy Peanut Caramel

# Slim•Fast Breakfast and Lunch Nutrition Bars

Dutch Chocolate
Peanut Butter

# Slim•Fast Meal On-The-Go Bars

Oatmeal Raisin            Rich Chocolate Brownie
Milk Chocolate Peanut     Apple Cobbler
Chocolate Cookie Dough    Honey Peanut
Toasted Oats & Spice

# Getting Your Portions Under Control

Let's face it: It's virtually impossible to count every calorie you consume, so most of the time you need to estimate how much you're eating. Knowing how to eyeball standard serving sizes will help you keep portions under control. Not sure what 3 ounces of chicken looks like? Or a teaspoon of margarine? Use this handy guide to take a quick measure of portion sizes:

| | |
|---|---|
| Fist | About 1 cup, or 1 medium fruit |
| Palm(minus fingers) | About 3 ounces cooked poultry, fish, or lean meat |
| Cupped hand | About 1 to 2 ounces pretzels (15 small twists, 7 regular) |
| Thumb | About 1 ounce cheese or meat |
| Thumbtip | About 1 tablespoon |
| Fingertip | About 1 teaspoon |

# Sensible Snacks

Making smart snack choices will give you energy during the day, help satisfy your appetite, and help you reach your weight-loss goal. Snacking on fresh fruits and vegetables will give you the most nutrition in the fewest amount of calories. Still, sometimes you may want to snack on something a little more substantial. Here are some healthy snacks that won't sabotage your weight-loss efforts. Enjoy two snacks from the 60- to 90-calorie category and one from the 100- to 150-calorie category each day.

## 60 to 90 Calories

1 piece fresh fruit
¾ cup blueberries
4 ounces fruit juice
¼ ounce pretzels, fat free
2 cups air-popped popcorn
6 saltine-type crackers
¾ ounce snack chips, fat free

8 animal crackers
3 graham crackers
1 ounce dried apricot snacks
¾-ounce packet apple chips
2 breadsticks
½ cup light fruit cocktail

## 100 to 150 Calories

1 Slim•Fast Snack Bar
1 cup nonfat yogurt
½ bagel with 1 tablespoon
   all-fruit spread
1 cup low-fat soup
½ cup frozen nonfat yogurt
½ cup low-fat ice milk
½ cup fat-free pudding

6 vanilla wafers
4 slices light rye crispbread
1 medium banana
1½ ounces mozzarella cheese
½ cup fruit sorbet
1 slice angel food cake
1 cup low-fat soup

# Your Weekly Shopping List

How many times have you had to forgo trying a new recipe because you were missing a few essential ingredients? You'll see that it pays to plan ahead and outline a weekly menu for yourself. Look over the breakfast, lunch, and dinner recipes on the following pages and think about what you want to prepare for the upcoming week. Check your kitchen for what you already have, then compose a shopping list with all the ingredients you'll need to get on your next trip to the supermarket. To help you stay organized, divide the list into the following categories:

Meat/Fish/Poultry     Dairy Products
Fruits and Vegetables     Spices
Beans and Legumes     Slim•Fast shakes and bars
Grains, Breads, Pasta     Miscellaneous

# Guide to Supermarket Shopping

Here's one thing you should know: Your supermarket shopping habits can make or break your weight-loss goals. The simple lessons you've always heard still hold: Never shop when you're hungry. Shop with a food list. And don't buy your favorite binge foods "for the family," because you'll end up eating them, too. As you're composing your shopping list, move mentally through the aisles and think about what's available in every section. Divide your list into sections and consider the pros and cons of the possibilities that await you.

### PRODUCE

Gazing upon row after row of brilliantly hued fruits and vegetables, give in to the temptation to try a new variety of tomato or an oddly shaped squash. This is the only area of the supermarket where it pays to be decadent. Getting a colorful array of fruits and vegetables will give you a greater variety of phytochemicals. And here's a surprise: Frozen or canned vegetables usually contain just as many vitamins and nutrients as their fresh counterparts.

Don't hurry through this section. Allow yourself time to inspect the produce, seeing what looks good and is on sale. Produce items won't break your budget and are ideal for boosting your health and your weight-loss efforts. And don't forget to load up on fresh vegetables at the salad bar—a great time-saver for lunch and dinner, if you don't mind paying a dollar or two more.

**Best choices:** Fill your basket with seasonal produce—it's freshest and cheapest. Here are just a few seasonal suggestions:

*Spring:* red peppers, fresh herbs (dill, basil, mint, etc.), carrots, yellow squash, spinach, pears, apricots, strawberries, mushrooms, eggplant, tomatoes

*Summer:* tomatoes, peaches, plums, nectarines, cherries, raspberries, blueberries, strawberries, yellow squash, fresh herbs, watermelon

*Fall:* apples, pears, carrots, onions, potatoes, cabbage, zucchini

*Winter:* Oranges, lemons, zucchini, carrots, onions, celery, red and green peppers, bananas, apples, pears, potatoes, cabbage

## CANNED AND PACKAGED GOODS

Spend the least amount of time in these center aisles, where the processed foods beckon. You'll find eye-catching packaging and sale items begging you to "buy and save," but don't be tempted into buying what you don't need. Steer clear of overly processed meal "kits," like a deli lunch-in-a-box or pizza and taco kits. These shortcuts are often loaded with sodium, fat, and calories, and most can be made nearly as quickly with fresh ingredients.

**Best choices:** Try this strategy: Leave your cart at the end of the aisle and grab only what you need and bring it back. This will keep you from throwing in cookies, chips, and boxed macaroni and cheese. In general, buy things as minimally processed as possible: low-sodium, whole-grain, high-fiber items. Some suggestions:

| | |
|---|---|
| Slow-cooked oatmeal | Salsa |
| Fat-free pretzels | Canned and dried beans |
| Melba toast | Couscous, polenta, or risotto |
| Reduced-calorie air-popped popcorn | Stewed tomatoes |
| | Low-fat crackers |
| Rice cakes | Canned salmon |
| Graham crackers | Canned vegetables (green beans, sweet potatoes, corn, etc.) |
| Dry cereal (with 5 grams fiber or more per serving) | |
| | Water-packed tuna |
| Low-fat bean dips | Slim•Fast shakes, snack bars, and meal bars |
| Whole-grain/brown rice | |

## MEATS, FISH, AND POULTRY

You can save money if you buy these pricier items when they're on sale or in larger quantities. Set aside what you need over the next two or three days, and freeze the rest.

**Best Choices:** Choose meats with the smallest amount of visible fat. Boneless roasts, chops, and skinless poultry may be more expensive, but throw off less waste. To get the freshest fish, ask if the fish was delivered that day or (at the latest) the day before. Don't rule out frozen cuts. If there's no sign of dryness (or ice crystals, which can indicate thawing), they're often fresher and cheaper than what's in the glass case. Some suggestions:

| | |
|---|---|
| Beef top round (Select) | Tuna steak |
| Skinless chicken breast | Turkey breast roast |
| Salmon steak | Flounder |
| Eye round (Select) | Extra-lean ground beef |
| Ground chicken or turkey | Turkey cutlets |
| (white meat) | Fillet of sole |

## THE DELI COUNTER AND PACKAGED MEATS

You'll need to navigate this area very carefully. Use restraint, and don't buy anything swimming in mayonnaise or oil. Don't be fooled into thinking that pasta salads, tuna salad, and oily vegetables are "salads" in the healthy sense of the word. They are havens for hidden fat and calories. Ditto for the meat loaf, stuffed peppers, and other prepared dishes that may tempt you with their ease and convenience. (Save the hidden calories for those special occasions when you dine out in restaurants.) Better deli choices include:

*Roasted or rotisserie chicken:* Peel off skin and slice into serving-size portions.

*Reduced-fat or fat-free lunch meat, roast beef, or turkey breast:* Get it thinly sliced and stick to the least processed choices (turkey breast rather than turkey loaf, for example).

*Reduced-fat hot dogs:* In general, poultry-based dogs are the leanest, but check the label for fat and calorie content. Anything marked "fat-free" is a great option, from hot dogs to sausages to bacon.

*Soy meats:* Ground beef, hot dogs, and burgers made from soy are a great option once you get used to the slight difference in taste. They're usually low in fat and packed with protein.

## FROZEN FOODS

It's easy to be seduced by the ice cream, cakes, and pies stacked in these aisles. Bypass them for these better options:

*Frozen vegetables:* Stock your freezer with frozen veggies so they're always on hand. Buy variety packs of three or more vegetables like broccoli, corn, carrots, and green beans—an easy way to get a few servings of vegetables with dinner. Also keep some boxes of frozen chopped spinach and broccoli on hand to mix into lasagna, meat loaf, and casseroles.

*Frozen fruit and fat-free sorbet:* Unsweetened frozen fruit can make a great dessert, or can be pureed into a quick sauce. Fat-free sorbets and fruit-juice Popsicles are great low-calorie snack options.

*Fat-free frozen yogurt and ice cream:* If you can find a brand and flavor that you like, these are great calorie-savers for a dessert or snack. Make sure you stick with serving-size portions, though—don't take the fat-free label as a license to overeat.

*Frozen dinner entrées:* These can be great time-savers if you don't have time to prepare your own dinner. Look for low-fat, vegetable-heavy entrées like Healthy Choice or Lean Cuisine. On the Slim•Fast Plan, you should be eating about around 600 calories for dinner, so you may need to eat two of these entrées to get a full meal.

## DAIRY

You'll be greeted with a plethora of choices from gourmet cheese to yogurts in every flavor. Supermarkets hope you'll be dazzled into buying products you don't really need. One rule of thumb: Don't buy cheeses to snack on or serve as an appetizer—you don't need the extra fat or calories before your meal. Some sensible picks:

*Low-fat dairy products:* Stock up on fat-free milk to use for cereal, low-fat cream sauces, and in Slim•Fast shakes. Diet margarine, no-calorie butter sprays, low-fat ricotta, and reduced-fat or fat-free cheeses are great lower-calorie options.

*Full-flavored cheeses (Parmesan and Roquefort):* These can be used as a flavoring or topping, and you only need to add a little bit to get the desired taste.

*Nonfat yogurt, sour cream, cottage cheese:* Fat-free or low-fat options will save you on calories. Go for the plain, unflavored versions to get the most versatility. You can cut your own fresh fruit into cottage cheese, use fresh herbs to make a tasty yogurt dip for your vegetables, and use sour cream to flavor baked potatoes.

*Cholesterol-free egg substitutes:* Add these to cake mixes and casseroles, or make your own vegetable omelet by stirring in some fresh peppers and mushrooms. They're an easy, convenient way to save on fat and calories.

## BAKERY

The bakery aisle offers too many goodies, and the smells of freshly baked cakes can be spellbinding. Still, there are healthy items here—if you keep your nose plugs on and your eyes focused on your list.

*High-fiber bread:* "Whole wheat" doesn't necessarily mean "high-fiber," nor do phrases like "rye," "whole grain," or "all-natural ingredients." The only way to tell if a bread is high in nutritious fiber is to read the label. Make sure each slice contains 3 grams or more of fiber. Also, look for brands that are reduced-calorie, so you can have two slices of bread for the same number of calories as one.

*Low-fat English muffins:* They're versatile. You can top them with tomato sauce and cheese, scrambled eggs, or raspberry preserves. Look for brands that are reduced-fat.

*Light dinner rolls:* These are good accompaniments with dinner. Look for brands with at least 3 grams of fiber per roll (and 100 calories or less).

*Angel food cake:* If you need a splurge, this isn't a bad option, since it's low in fat and calories. Still, watch your portions. Buy the cake if you must, but cut it into serving-size pieces when you get home and freeze each individually.

# The Recipes

*A note on packaged soups and salad dressings:* Many brands of commercially pre-pared low-fat soups and salad dressings are available on store shelves. When shopping for these items, look carefully at the Nutrition Facts panel. For *low-fat soups,* select those with 3 grams or less of fat per serving, with 1 gram or less saturated fat. Also, look at sodium content, which is often very high in canned soups. Look for "healthy" low-fat varieties with 475 mg or less of sodium per serving.

Commercial salad dressings are available as reduced-fat, lite, low-calorie, and fat-free. Look for those with 0 grams of saturated fat per serving (serving size is 2 tablespoons). Again, sodium content may often be very high; however, there are brands available with lower sodium content that are fat-free *and* flavorful.

# Discovering the Kitchen

A great gift this Slim•Fast life has given me is . . . the art of cooking! I've always *wanted* to cook well, and I've often fooled myself into thinking I knew what I was doing—at least until an Italian painter friend of mine teased me once: "Lauren, you *act* cooking."

Well, you can only get away with acting for so long (at least until you have to throw a dinner party). So now, after a Creamy Milk Chocolate breakfast and lunch, by dinner I'm ready to *eat*. And I'm not taking any chances on messing anything up. For the first time in my life, I'm following recipes closely—and creating some of my own! No more half-baked shortcuts, no more talking on the phone or wandering off to read a book midstream. Now I stick to the business at hand—and the results are delicious.

And when I get a sudden urge to cook in the *middle* of the day, I'm always able to throw together some terrific salsa, or relish, or my beloved tabouleh. Give me lots of tomatoes to chop, jalapeños, Italian parsley, red onions, and mint, and I'm happy.

Now, I love hot stuff—especially dishes made with jalapeños or habaneros (Scotch bonnet peppers). Jalapeños are usually mildly hot, depending on how many you use in a dish, but habaneros—fasten your seat belts. I eat pickled jalapeños whole, like candy; I used to order them by the case from Steve's in Dallas, Texas. A small slice of one tiny Scotch bonnet, on the other hand, is all I can handle, but the flavor is indescribable. Try either of them in salsas or relishes—just be careful if you're a beginner!

# Stocking the Kitchen

Now that I've become so much more interested in cooking, here's a quick sketch of all the wonderful things I keep on hand in my kitchen *at all times*—a host of great foodstuffs and fixings that makes it easy to eat healthy every day.

Filter pitcher full of water

Raw (unprocessed) apple and cranberry juice

Red grapefruit

The berries—blue, black, rasp

Lemons and limes

Cucumbers

Broccoli

Organic tomatoes and plum tomatoes

Yellow and spaghetti squash

Carrots

Celery

Radishes

Bean sprouts

Sweet Bermuda onions

Red onions

Habaneros (Scotch bonnets)

Jalapeños

Shiitake mushrooms

Lettuce (any kind)

Fresh spinach

Endive

Italian parsley

Cilantro

Scallions

Shallots

Fresh gingerroot

Fresh horseradish

Tons of garlic

Firm tofu

Pasta in all varieties (I buy the fresh varieties—find them in your grocer's dairy section)

Low-sodium chicken broth

Rice: brown and basmati

Bulgur wheat

Polenta

Dried beans: split pea; green and yellow; cannellini; black and red (pinto); fragolinis; kidneys

Wild white sage honey

Every spice I can get my hands on—whole or powdered. Buy in small bulk, and bottle them yourself; don't forget to replace them if they get too old (after a year or so)

Low-fat flour or corn tortillas

Black olive paste

Sweet pepper paste

Good Parmesan cheese (whole, not pregrated)

Extra-virgin olive oil

White peach and mint tea

Six-pack of Slim•Fast in the fridge

A few other things I keep around the kitchen:

Stone mortar and pestle (for grinding spices, etc.)
Half-moon double-bladed knife (for chopping)
Knife sharpener
Thick hardwood chopping block
Toaster oven for tortillas
Coffee grinder
Food processor
Spinning spice rack (sixteen bottles in a five-inch square!)

# The Recipes

## Chicken and Turkey

**Warm Chicken and Vegetable Salad**

●

**Mediterranean Chicken Pockets**

●

**Chicken and Fettuccine Dijon**

●

**Honey-Grilled Chicken Breast**

●

**Grilled Turkey Kabobs in Pita**

●

**Turkey Fajitas**

●

**Turkey Cutlets with Cranberry Sauce**

---

Warm Chicken and Vegetable Salad
Sautéed Portobello Mushrooms
Whole wheat crackers
Cantaloupe wedge

# Warm Chicken and Vegetable Salad

*Total preparation time: 60 minutes*

2 large Idaho potatoes, scrubbed well, peeled, and sliced 1 inch thick
1 pound fresh green beans, trimmed, washed, and cut into 2-inch pieces
Nonstick cooking spray
1¾ pounds boneless, skinless chicken breasts, washed, dried,
   and cut into 2-inch pieces
2 large tomatoes, washed and quartered
1 small red onion, peeled and diced
½ cup fat-free mayonnaise
1 tablespoon lemon juice
½ teaspoon thyme
½ teaspoon tarragon
¼ teaspoon salt
½ teaspoon pepper
1 head romaine lettuce, outer leaves removed, washed, dried,
   and leaves separated

1. Fill a large saucepan with enough water to cover potatoes and set to boil. Add potatoes to boiling water, reduce heat to medium, and cook 15 to 20 minutes, until tender when pierced with a fork. Drain, cool, and dice.
2. Meanwhile, fill a medium saucepan with 2 inches water and set to boil. Put cut green beans in steamer or colander, place in saucepan, and steam 5 minutes, or until crisp-tender.
3. Spray a large nonstick skillet with cooking spray and warm over medium heat. Add chicken and sauté 5 to 8 minutes, turning frequently, until thoroughly cooked and no longer pink inside.
4. In a large mixing bowl, combine cooked chicken, diced potatoes, steamed green beans, tomato quarters, and diced onion. Add mayonnaise, lemon juice, thyme, tarragon, salt, and pepper, and blend well.
5. Place lettuce leaves on serving plates. Top with warm chicken and vegetable mixture, and serve with 4 whole-wheat crackers per portion.

SERVES 4

# Sautéed Portobello Mushrooms

*Total preparation time: 15 minutes*

**Nonstick cooking spray**
**1 pound portobello mushrooms, rinsed, dried, and cut into**
   **½ -inch-thick slices**
**3 tablespoons Worcestershire sauce**
**½ teaspoon ground black pepper**
**¼ cup chopped parsley**

Spray a large nonstick skillet with cooking spray. Add mushrooms and Worcestershire sauce and sauté 5 to 7 minutes over medium heat, until mushrooms are soft. Add pepper and parsley and cook 2 to 3 minutes. Drain excess moisture, remove to a platter, and serve.

SERVES 4

NUTRITIONAL INFORMATION PER SERVING

|  | Calories | Protein | Carbohydrates | Fat | Fiber | Sodium | Cholesterol | Calcium |
|---|---|---|---|---|---|---|---|---|
| **Warm Chicken Salad** | 487 | 55 g | 36 g | 14 g | 6 g | 491 mg | 143 mg | 98 mg |
| **Sautéed Portobello Mushrooms** | 42 | 4 g | 6 g | 2 g | 2 g | 132 mg | 0 mg | 23 mg |
| **4 whole-wheat crackers** | 71 | 1.5 g | 11 g | 3 g | 2 g | 105 mg | 0 mg | 8 mg |
| **Cantaloupe wedge (¹/₈ melon)** | 24 | 1 g | 6 g | 0.5 g | 0.5 g | 6 mg | 0 mg | 8 mg |
| **Meal Total** | 624 | 61.5 g | 59 g | 19 g (27%)* | 10.5 g | 734 mg | 143 mg | 137 mg |

*Percentage of calories from fat

---

Mediterranean Chicken Pockets
Quick Carrot Slaw
Grapes

---

# Mediterranean Chicken Pockets

*Total preparation time: 20 minutes*

Nonstick cooking spray
1 teaspoon canola oil
1½ pounds boneless, skinless chicken breasts
One 10-ounce box frozen peas
2 medium tomatoes, washed and chopped
2 ounces feta cheese, crumbled
1 scallion, washed, trimmed, and chopped
½ cup plain nonfat yogurt
½ cup fat-free mayonnaise
1 tablespoon lemon juice
1 teaspoon dried dillweed
Four 1½-ounce pita bread rounds, halved crosswise
½ small head iceberg lettuce, outer leaves removed, washed,
    dried, and separated into leaves

1.  Spray a large nonstick skillet with cooking spray, brush with oil, and heat over medium-high flame. Add chicken breasts and sauté, turning frequently, until cooked and no longer pink inside, 8 to 10 minutes, or until internal temperature is 170°F. Remove from skillet, place on platter, cover, and let cool in refrigerator.
2.  Meanwhile, bring ½ cup water to boil in a medium saucepan, and add frozen peas. Bring to a boil, reduce heat, cover, and simmer 4 minutes; do not overcook. Drain and set aside.

3.  Cut cooled chicken into ½-inch pieces. In a large bowl, combine chicken, cooked peas, tomatoes, feta cheese, and scallion. Fold in yogurt, mayonnaise, lemon juice, and dillweed, and toss well.
4.  Line inside of pita halves with lettuce and stuff with chicken mixture.

SERVES 4

# Quick Carrot Slaw

*Total preparation time: 10 to 12 minutes*

**4 large carrots, ends removed, peeled, and shredded**
**1 small red onion, peeled and thinly sliced**
**¼ cup apple cider or apple juice**
**2 tablespoons reduced-fat mayonnaise**
**2 tablespoons cider vinegar**
**½ teaspoon sugar substitute**
**¼ teaspoon salt**
**¼ teaspoon ground pepper**

*Food-processor method:* Combine all ingredients in food processor, and pulse 4 or 5 times until all ingredients are finely chopped and blended together. *Hand method:* After shredding carrot and slicing onion, chop very finely. Place all ingredients in medium mixing bowl and stir until well-blended. Transfer to a serving bowl, cover, and chill before serving.

SERVES 4

NUTRITIONAL INFORMATION PER SERVING

|  | Calories | Protein | Carbohydrate | Fat | Fiber | Sodium | Cholesterol | Calcium |
|---|---|---|---|---|---|---|---|---|
| **Mediterranean Chicken Pockets** | 519 | 49 g | 46 g | 15 g | 6 g | 794 mg | 116 mg | 206 mg |
| **Quick Carrot Slaw** | 85 | 1.5 g | 18 g | 2 g | 4 g | 223 mg | 2 mg | 38 mg |
| **Grapes (about 15)** | 53 | 0.5 g | 13 g | 0.5 g | 1 g | 2 mg | 0 mg | 8 mg |
| **Meal Total** | 657 | 51 g | 77 g | 17 g (23%) | 11 g | 1,019 mg | 118 mg | 252 mg |

Chicken and Fettuccine Dijon
Rosemary-Steamed Broccoli and Carrots
Tossed Salad with Tomatoes
Medium fresh orange

## Chicken and Fettuccine Dijon

*Total preparation time: 20 to 25 minutes*

1 cup fat-free sour cream
1½ tablespoons Dijon-style mustard
½ teaspoon dried thyme
Four 7-ounce boneless, skinless chicken breasts
Nonstick cooking spray
½ pound button mushrooms, washed, dried, and thinly sliced
2 tablespoons water
6 ounces fettuccine
½ lemon, sliced very thin
½ teaspoon freshly ground black pepper

1.  In a small bowl, stir together sour cream, mustard, and thyme.
2.  Rinse chicken and pat dry. Spray a large nonstick skillet with cooking spray. Place on medium heat and add chicken. Sauté, stirring frequently, 8 to 10 minutes, or until chicken is cooked through and no longer pink. Remove chicken from skillet, place on platter, and cover to keep warm. Add mushrooms with 2 tablespoons water into skillet, cover, and cook over medium heat until soft, about 2 minutes. Add sour-cream mixture to mushrooms and heat, but do not boil. Return chicken to skillet and gently mix with mushroom and sour cream sauce.

3.  Meanwhile, bring 6 cups of water to boil in a large pot. Add fettuccine and cook, stirring frequently, until al dente (firm to the bite), 6 to 7 minutes or according to package directions. Remove from heat, drain, set aside, and keep warm.

4.  Place warm fettuccine on a serving platter and top with chicken and sauce. Garnish with lemon slices and sprinkle with freshly ground pepper.

SERVES 4

## Tossed Salad with Tomatoes

*Total preparation time: 10 to 12 minutes*

½ **head romaine lettuce, outer leaves removed, washed, dried, and torn into bite-size pieces**

½ **head iceberg lettuce, outer leaves removed, washed, dried, and torn into bite-size pieces**

**4 medium tomatoes, washed and cut into small wedges**

½ **cup fat-free salad dressing**

Place lettuce in a large salad bowl and toss with tomato wedges. Dress immediately before serving.

SERVES 4

# Rosemary–Steamed Broccoli and Carrots

*Total preparation time: 12 minutes*

1 tablespoon chopped fresh rosemary or 1 teaspoon dried
2 pounds broccoli, rinsed, stems and rough ends removed, cut into bite-size
    flowerets
1 pound fresh carrots, tops and bottoms removed, peeled, washed, and
    sliced into ¼-inch pieces

Fill a large saucepan with 2 inches water and set to boil. Add chopped rosemary to water and reduce heat to simmer. Place broccoli and carrots in a steaming basket or colander over water and steam 5 minutes, or until crisp-tender.

SERVES 4

### NUTRITIONAL INFORMATION PER SERVING

| | Calories | Protein | Carbohydrate | Fat | Fiber | Sodium | Cholesterol | Calcium |
|---|---|---|---|---|---|---|---|---|
| **Chicken and Fettuccine Dijon** | 450 | 57 g | 40 g | 5.5 g | 2 g | 331 mg | 154 mg | 128 mg |
| **Rosemary-Steamed Broccoli and Carrots** | 89 | 5 g | 19 g | 1 g | 8 g | 77 mg | 0 mg | 103 mg |
| **Tossed Salad with Tomatoes** | 70 | 3 g | 15 g | 1 g | 4 g | 38 mg | 0 mg | 52 mg |
| **Medium fresh orange** | 62 | 1 g | 15 g | 0 g | 3 g | 0 mg | 0 mg | 52 mg |
| **Meal Total** | 671 | 66 g | 89 g | 7.5 g (10%) | 17 g | 446 mg | 154 mg | 335 mg |

Honey-Grilled Chicken Breast
Tossed Salad
Sliced apple with cinnamon
Baked Sweet Potato
Oregano-Scented Summer Squash
Steamed Spinach
Parsley Carrot Coins

# Honey-Grilled Chicken Breast

*Total preparation time: 45 minutes*

**1 tablespoon orange juice**
**2 teaspoons lemon juice**
**2 teaspoons honey**
**2 teaspoons light (reduced-sodium) soy sauce**
**1 teaspoon grated fresh gingerroot**
**1 clove garlic, peeled and minced**
**Four 7-ounce boneless, skinless chicken breasts**

1.  Combine all ingredients except chicken in large shallow dish and whisk until blended. Add chicken breasts, turn several times to coat, cover with plastic wrap, and set in refrigerator. Marinate 15 minutes or up to 1 hour.
2.  Meanwhile, prepare outdoor grill.
3.  Grill the chicken breasts 3 inches from heat 4 to 5 minutes per side, or until cooked through and juices run clear, or internal temperature is 170°F.
4.  Remove to a plate and let stand 5 minutes before serving.

SERVES 4

# Tossed Salad

*Total preparation time: 10 minutes*

1 small head romaine lettuce, outer leaves removed, washed, dried, and torn
   into bite-size pieces
1 small head red-leaf lettuce, outer leaves removed, washed, dried, and torn
   into bite-size pieces
2 dozen cherry tomatoes, rinsed and halved
1 small red onion, peeled and thinly sliced
12 button mushrooms, washed, dried, and thinly sliced
½ cup fat-free salad dressing

Toss all ingredients except dressing in a large salad bowl. Dress immediately before serving.

SERVES 4

# Baked Sweet Potato

*Total preparation time: 5 to 8 or 50 to 60 minutes, depending on method*

2 medium sweet potatoes, with skin (see Note), scrubbed well, ends
   trimmed

*Oven method:* Preheat oven to 400°F. Prick potatoes a few times with a fork. Place on baking sheet and bake 50 to 60 minutes, or until soft when pierced by a fork. *Microwave method:* Prick potatoes twice with a fork. Place side by side on a paper towel in center of microwave oven. Cook on high 5 to 8 minutes, or until soft when pierced by a fork.

SERVES 4
Note: The skin of sweet potatoes contains many nutrients and fiber and should be left on and eaten whenever possible.

## Oregano–Scented Summer Squash

*Total preparation time: 10 minutes*

**1 teaspoon dried *or* 1 tablespoon fresh chopped oregano**
**1 pound yellow summer squash, tops and bottoms removed, washed, and**
**　　cut into ½-inch slices**

Fill a large saucepan with 2 inches water and set to boil. Add oregano. Place summer squash in steamer or colander and place in saucepan. Steam 5 minutes, or until crisp-tender.

SERVES 4

## Steamed Spinach

*Total preparation time: 10 minutes*

**2 pounds fresh spinach, tough ends removed, washed thoroughly**

Fill a large saucepan with 2 inches water and set to boil. Place spinach in steamer or colander and place in saucepan. Steam spinach 5 minutes, or until wilted but still bright green.

SERVES 4

## Parsley Carrot Coins

*Total preparation time: 15 minutes*

**1 pound carrots, peeled, trimmed, and cut into ¼-inch slices**
**2 tablespoons chopped fresh parsley**

Fill a large saucepan with 2 inches water and set to boil. Place carrots in steamer or colander and place in saucepan. Steam 8 to 10 minutes, or until crisp-tender. Toss with parsley and serve.

SERVES 4

NUTRITIONAL INFORMATION PER SERVING

|  | Calories | Protein | Carbohydrate | Fat | Fiber | Sodium | Cholesterol | Calcium |
|---|---|---|---|---|---|---|---|---|
| Honey-Grilled Chicken Breast | 298 | 43 g | 4 g | 11 g | 0 g | 202 mg | 120 mg | 23 mg |
| Tossed Salad | 88 | 5 g | 18 g | 1 g | 5 g | 35 mg | 0 mg | 73 mg |
| Baked Sweet Potato | 59 | 1 g | 14 g | 0 g | 2 g | 6 mg | 0 mg | 16 mg |
| Oregano-Scented Summer Squash | 23 | 1 g | 5 g | 0 g | 2 g | 2 mg | 0 mg | 27 mg |
| Steamed Spinach | 36 | 5 g | 6 g | 0.5 g | 4 g | 129 mg | 0 mg | 162 mg |
| Parsley Carrot Coins | 49 | 1 g | 12 g | 0 | 3 g | 41 mg | 0 mg | 33 mg |
| sliced apple (1 medium) | 81 | 0 g | 21 g | 0.5 g | 4 g | 0 mg | 0 mg | 10 mg |
| Meal Total | 634 | 56 g | 89 g | 13 g (18%) | 20 g | 415 mg | 120 mg | 344 mg |

**Grilled Turkey Kabobs in Pita**
**Cucumber–Yogurt Salad**
**Nectarine**

# Grilled Turkey Kabobs in Pita

*Total preparation time: 1 hour*

1 tablespoon minced fresh dill
1 teaspoon dried oregano
4 cloves garlic, peeled and minced
$\frac{1}{4}$ teaspoon ground black pepper
1$\frac{3}{4}$ pounds turkey breast tenders, cut into 2-inch cubes
3 large yellow onions, peeled and cut into wedges
3 large tomatoes, washed and cut into wedges
12 large button mushrooms, washed, dried, and halved
Four 6$\frac{1}{2}$-inch pita bread pockets

1. Combine dill, oregano, garlic, and pepper in a small mixing bowl. Place turkey pieces in a shallow dish, sprinkle with half the spice mixture, and toss to coat. Cover, refrigerate, and marinate 15 minutes or up to 1 hour.
2. Prepare grill 20 minutes before preparation time, or preheat oven to 425°F.
3. In a medium mixing bowl, toss the remaining half of the spice mix with the onions, tomatoes, and mushrooms.
4. Prepare foil packets: using two large sheets of aluminum foil, place half the marinated turkey in the center of each, and surround with vegetables. Bring up the sides of the foil and double fold. Then double fold the ends to form a packet, leaving 2 inches on each end for heat circulation.
5. Grill, covered, 20 minutes, or bake on a cookie sheet in 425°F oven 25 minutes.
6. Split pita rounds in half, and serve grilled kabobs on bread.

SERVES 4

# Cucumber–Yogurt Salad

*Total preparation time: 30 to 60 minutes*

**4 medium cucumbers, peeled and thinly sliced**
**1 teaspoon salt**
**2 cups plain nonfat yogurt**
**1 head red- or green-leaf lettuce, outer leaves removed, washed, dried, and
  shredded**

1. Place sliced cucumbers in a large mixing bowl and add salt. Mix and let stand 5 minutes.
2. With a paper towel, pat cucumbers dry. Add yogurt and toss well to coat. Cover and refrigerate 15 minutes or up to 45 minutes.
3. Arrange lettuce leaves on individual plates and top with cucumber mixture.

SERVES 4

NUTRITIONAL INFORMATION PER SERVING

| | Calories | Protein | Carbohydrate | Fat | Fiber | Sodium | Cholesterol | Calcium |
|---|---|---|---|---|---|---|---|---|
| Grilled Turkey Kabobs in Pita | 471 | 60 g | 50 g | 3 g | 5 g | 426 mg | 141 mg | 122 mg |
| Cucumber-Yogurt Salad | 94 | 8 g | 19 g | 0.5 g | 3 g | 657 mg | 3 mg | 205 mg |
| Nectarine (1 medium) | 66 | 1 g | 16 g | 1 g | 2 g | 0 mg | 0 mg | 7 mg |
| Meal Total | 631 | 69 g | 85 g | 4.5 (13%) | 10 g | 1,083 mg | 144 mg | 334 mg |

Turkey Fajitas
Mixed Green Salad (page 198)
Sliced papaya

# Turkey Fajitas

*Total preparation time: 20 minutes*

Nonstick cooking spray
1¾ pounds turkey tender strips
4 teaspoons olive oil
4 cloves garlic, peeled and minced
2 medium yellow onions, peeled and thinly sliced
1 medium red pepper, washed, cored, seeded, and sliced into strips
1 medium green pepper, washed, cored, seeded, and sliced into strips
½ teaspoon cumin
¼ teaspoon coriander
1 teaspoon oregano
1 teaspoon paprika
¼ teaspoon red cayenne pepper

¾ teaspoon chili powder

4 tablespoons nonfat sour cream

4 medium low-fat flour or corn tortillas (see Note)

½ cup salsa

¼ cup shredded fat-free Monterey Jack cheese

1.  Spray a large nonstick skillet with cooking spray. Place over medium heat, add turkey strips, and sauté 5 to 8 minutes, turning frequently, until thoroughly cooked and no longer pink inside.
2.  Remove turkey from skillet and set aside, covered. Add olive oil, garlic, and onions to skillet. Sauté over medium heat until garlic is golden and onions translucent, 3 to 5 minutes.
3.  Add red and green pepper strips, cumin, coriander, oregano, paprika, cayenne, and chili powder. Continue to cook until peppers are wilted but still crisp, 5 to 6 minutes.
4.  Return cooked turkey strips to vegetable mixture and gently mix.
5.  Spread nonfat sour cream on top of warm tortillas. Divide fajita mixture among the 4 tortillas and top each with 1 tablespoon salsa and 1 tablespoon cheese. Roll and serve warm.

SERVES 4

Note: To warm tortillas in the microwave, place flat in microwave and heat on medium 45 to 50 seconds until hot; do not overheat. Oven method: Wrap tortillas in aluminum foil and warm in 250°F oven 10 minutes.

NUTRITIONAL INFORMATION PER SERVING

|  | Calories | Protein | Carbohydrate | Fat | Fiber | Sodium | Cholesterol | Calcium |
|---|---|---|---|---|---|---|---|---|
| **Turkey Fajitas** | 591 | 53 g | 42 g | 22 g | 5 g | 577 mg | 130 mg | 221 mg |
| **Mixed Green Salad** | 115 | 6 g | 24 g | 1 g | 7 g | 44 mg | 0 mg | 131 mg |
| **Sliced papaya (1/2)** | 59 | 1 g | 15 g | 0 g | 3 g | 5 mg | 0 mg | 36 mg |
| **Meal Total** | 765 | 60 g | 81 g | 23 g (27%) | 15 g | 626 mg | 130 mg | 388 mg |

Turkey Cutlets with Cranberry Sauce
Wild Rice
Green Beans
Mashed Butternut Squash with Brown Sugar
Mixed Garden Salad (page 174)
Cantaloupe wedge

# Turkey Cutlets with Cranberry Sauce

*Total preparation time: 20 minutes*

Four 7-ounce turkey breast tenders
½ teaspoon ground nutmeg
½ cup fat-free chicken broth
1 tablespoon cornstarch
15 ounces (1 can) whole cranberry sauce

1.  Preheat broiler.
2.  Rinse turkey and pat dry. Sprinkle lightly with nutmeg.
3.  Place turkey on a broiler rack 4 to 5 inches from heat, and cook 7 minutes. Turn and cook 4 to 5 minutes more, until no longer pink and internal temperature is 170°F.
4.  Meanwhile, combine chicken broth and cornstarch in a small saucepan. Simmer over medium heat, stirring frequently, until bubbly and thickened. Add cranberry sauce and cook, stirring constantly, 2 minutes.
5.  Place broiled turkey cutlets on a platter, top with cranberry sauce, and serve.

SERVES 4

# Wild Rice

*Total preparation time: 1 hour*

**½ cup uncooked wild rice, rinsed**

In a heavy 2-quart saucepan, bring 4 cups of water to a boil. Add rice, reduce heat to very low, cover tightly, and simmer gently 30 minutes. Shut off heat and let stand on burner 25 to 30 minutes, until rice reaches desired texture. Drain completely and serve warm.

SERVES 4

# Green Beans

*Total preparation time: 15 minutes*

**1 pound fresh green beans, stringed, trimmed, washed, and cut into 2-inch pieces**

Fill a medium saucepan with 2 inches water and set to boil. Place cut green beans in steamer or colander and place in saucepan. Steam 5 minutes, or until crisp-tender.

SERVES 4

# Mashed Butternut Squash with Brown Sugar

*Total preparation time: 40 to 55 minutes*

2 medium butternut squash (about 1 pound), washed, cut in half, with
    seeds and stringy parts removed
1 tablespoon brown sugar
⅛ teaspoon ground nutmeg
⅛ teaspoon ground cinnamon
¼ teaspoon grated orange peel (orange part only, with no white pith)

1.   Preheat oven to 400°F.
2.   In a shallow baking dish, place squash halves cut-side down. Cover with
     foil and bake 30 to 45 minutes, or until flesh is tender when pierced with
     a fork.
3.   Remove from oven, peel, and cut into cubes.
4.   In a large bowl, combine cubed squash, brown sugar, nutmeg, cinnamon,
     and orange peel. Mash together or, using an electric mixer, beat on
     medium speed until fluffy.

SERVES 4

NUTRITIONAL INFORMATION PER SERVING

|  | *Calories* | *Protein* | *Carbohydrate* | *Fat* | *Fiber* | *Sodium* | *Cholesterol* | *Calcium* |
|---|---|---|---|---|---|---|---|---|
| **Turkey Cutlets with Cranberry Sauce** | 487 | 49 g | 42 g | 13 g | 2 g | 227 mg | 126 mg | 38 mg |
| **Wild Rice** | 80 | 3 g | 17 g | 0 g | 1 g | 2 mg | 0 mg | 2 mg |
| **Green Beans** | 34 | 2 g | 8 g | 0 g | 3 g | 3 mg | 0 mg | 45 mg |
| **Mashed Butternut Squash with Brown Sugar** | 57 | 1 g | 15 g | 0 g | 3 g | 5 mg | 0 mg | 50 mg |
| **Mixed Garden Salad** | 74 | 3 g | 16 g | 1 g | 4 g | 37 mg | 0 mg | 56 mg |
| **Cantaloupe** | 24 | 1 g | 6 g | 0 g | 0.5 g | 6 mg | 0 mg | 8 mg |
| **Meal Total** | 756 | 59 g | 104 g | 14 g (17%) | 13.5 g | 280 mg | 126 mg | 199 mg |

# Seafood

**Curried Tuna Salad**

●

**Broiled Salmon with Penne Primavera**

●

**Seafood Strata**

●

**Grilled Red Snapper with Charred Tomato Salsa**

●

**Herb-Rubbed Grilled Tuna**

●

**Balsamic-Grilled Halibut Steak**

●

**Lemon-Pepper Sole**

---

**Curried Tuna Salad**
**French bread**
**Vegetable juice**
**Vanilla low-fat yogurt with ginger snaps**

# Curried Tuna Salad

*Total preparation time: 20 minutes*

Three 6-ounce cans solid white albacore tuna packed in water, drained and
  flaked
One 16-ounce can unpeeled apricot halves, in juice, quartered
1 pint strawberries, washed, hulled, and thinly sliced
2 celery stalks, washed, trimmed, and finely diced
¼ cup fat-free mayonnaise
½ cup plain nonfat yogurt
½ teaspoon curry powder
2 tablespoons lemon juice
1 head red-leaf lettuce, outer leaves removed, washed and dried

1.  In a large bowl, combine tuna with apricots, sliced strawberries, and
    diced celery. Mix thoroughly.
2.  In a small bowl, blend mayonnaise with the yogurt, curry powder, and
    lemon juice. Line 4 dinner plates with lettuce leaves, spoon tuna mixture
    onto plates, and top with dressing.

SERVES 4

NUTRITIONAL INFORMATION PER SERVING

| | Calories | Protein | Carbohydrate | Fat | Fiber | Sodium | Cholesterol | Calcium |
|---|---|---|---|---|---|---|---|---|
| Curried Tuna Salad | 278 | 34 g | 27 g | 5 g | 5 g | 638 mg | 56 mg | 123 mg |
| French bread (1 ounce) | 78 | 3 g | 15 g | 1 g | 1 g | 173 mg | 0 mg | 21 mg |
| Vegetable juice (1 cup) | 60 | 2 g | 11 g | 0 g | 2 g | 140 mg | 0 mg | 40 mg |
| Vanilla low-fat yogurt (½ cup) | 105 | 6 g | 17 g | 1.5 g | 0 g | 81 mg | 6 mg | 209 mg |
| Gingersnaps (3 small) | 90 | 1 g | 16 g | 2 g | 0.5 g | 128 mg | 0 mg | 15 mg |
| Meal Total | 611 | 46 g | 86 g | 113 g | 8.5 g | 1,160 mg | 62 mg | 408 mg |

Tomato vegetable soup (ready–made)
Broiled Salmon with Penne Primavera
Mixed Garden Salad
Watermelon wedge

# Broiled Salmon with Penne Primavera

*Total preparation time: 20 minutes*

8 ounces penne pasta

4 teaspoons olive oil

4 large cloves garlic, peeled and minced *or* ½ teaspoon prepared minced
   garlic

1 head  broccoli, rough ends removed, washed, and cut into bite-size pieces

2 medium red peppers, washed, cored, seeded, and cut into ¼-inch-wide
   strips

8 large button mushrooms, washed, dried, and thinly sliced

1 large yellow onion, peeled, halved, and thinly sliced

Nonstick cooking spray

¼ cup lemon juice

Four 6-ounce salmon steaks *or* 1½ pounds salmon fillet

¼ cup grated Parmesan cheese

1. Bring 6 cups water to boil in a large pot. Add penne, stir occasionally, and cook 7 to 8 minutes or until al dente. Drain, set aside, and keep warm.
2. Meanwhile, heat 2 teaspoons oil in nonstick skillet over medium-high flame. Add garlic and sauté until golden, about 30 seconds. Add broccoli, peppers, mushrooms, and onion and sauté until tender, 5 to 7 minutes.
3. Preheat broiler. Spray broiler pan with cooking spray, and place salmon on it.

4.  In a small bowl, combine remaining olive oil with lemon juice. Brush on salmon, basting both sides. Broil 3 to 4 minutes on one side, turn, and broil 3 to 4 minutes more or until fish flakes easily with a fork. Place on platter and keep warm.

5.  In a large bowl, combine vegetable mixture with penne. Toss with grated Parmesan cheese. Serve immediately with salmon.

SERVES 4

# Mixed Garden Salad

*Total preparation time: 10 to 12 minutes*

1 small head Boston, Bibb, or red-leaf lettuce, outer leaves removed, washed, dried, and torn into bite-size pieces
10 ounces arugula, tough ends removed, washed, and dried
1 small red onion, peeled and thinly sliced
24 cherry tomatoes, washed and halved
½ cup fat-free salad dressing

Place lettuce in large salad bowl and toss with arugula, onion, and tomatoes. Dress immediately before serving.

SERVES 4

NUTRITIONAL INFORMATION PER SERVING

|  | Calories | Protein | Carbohydrate | Fat | Fiber | Sodium | Cholesterol | Calcium |
|---|---|---|---|---|---|---|---|---|
| **Tomato vegetable soup (1 cup)** | 80 | 6 g | 17 g | 0 g | 5 g | 240 mg | 0 mg | 40 mg |
| **Broiled Salmon with Penne Primavera** | 503 | 42 g | 29 g | 24 g | 4 g | 208 mg | 98 mg | 151 mg |
| **Mixed Garden Salad** | 74 | 3 g | 16 g | 1 g | 4 g | 37 mg | 0 mg | 56 mg |
| **Watermelon wedge (¹⁄₁₆ melon)** | 92 | 2 g | 21 g | 1 g | 1 g | 6 mg | 0 mg | 23 mg |
| **Meal Total** | 749 | 53 g | 83 g | 26 g | 14 g | 491 mg | 98 mg | 270 mg |

Seafood Strata
Asparagus Spears (page 226)
Parsley Carrot Coins (page 163)
Red Beets (page 227)
Multicolored Salad (page 218)
Fresh sweet cherries

## Seafood Strata

*Total preparation time: 95 minutes (see Note)*

4 slices day-old white bread
Nonstick cooking spray
½ teaspoon canola or olive oil
4 ounces button mushrooms, washed, ends trimmed, and thinly sliced
1 scallion, trimmed and diced
¼ cup dry sherry
½ pound imitation crabmeat (pollack)
¾ cup shredded reduced-fat Swiss cheese
½ cup egg substitute
¾ cup 1% milk
⅛ teaspoon salt
⅛ teaspoon ground white pepper
1 medium tomato, thinly sliced
1 tablespoon chopped fresh chives

1. Preheat oven to 375°F.
2. Trim crusts from bread, place on ungreased baking sheet, and bake 10 minutes, until lightly browned. Reduce heat to 350°F.

3.  Spray a large nonstick skillet with cooking spray, brush with oil, and set over medium-high heat. Add mushrooms and sauté 10 minutes, turning occasionally, until liquid has evaporated. Add scallion and sauté 1 to 2 minutes. Add sherry, bring to a boil, and cook 1 minute. Reduce heat to low, add imitation crabmeat, mix well, and remove from heat; set aside.

4.  Spray an 8 x 8-inch glass or ceramic baking dish with vegetable cooking spray. Place 2 slices of the toasted bread in the dish, sprinkle with half the cheese, and top with the imitation crabmeat mixture. Top with the remaining 2 slices of bread and sprinkle with the remaining cheese.

5.  In a large bowl, beat egg substitute with milk, salt, and pepper. Pour egg mixture over top of bread, distributing evenly. Top with tomato slices.

6.  Bake in 350°F oven 45 to 50 minutes, or until knife inserted in center comes out clean. Let stand 10 minutes. Garnish with chopped chives and serve.

SERVES 4

Note: This strata can be assembled the day before, refrigerated, and baked the next day.

NUTRITIONAL INFORMATION PER SERVING

|  | Calories | Protein | Carbohydrate | Fat | Fiber | Sodium | Cholesterol | Calcium |
|---|---|---|---|---|---|---|---|---|
| **Seafood Strata** | 277 | 22 g | 24 g | 9 g | 1 g | 456 mg | 84 mg | 349 mg |
| **Asparagus Spears** | 39 | 4 g | 8 g | 0.5 g | 3.5 g | 3 mg | 0 mg | 36 mg |
| **Parsley Carrot Coins** | 49 | 1 g | 12 g | 0 g | 3 g | 41 mg | 0 mg | 33 mg |
| **Red Beets** | 75 | 3 g | 17 g | 0 g | 1 g | 122 mg | 0 mg | 27 mg |
| **Multicolored Salad** | 85 | 3 g | 18 g | 1 g | 3 g | 78 mg | 0 mg | 127 mg |
| **Fresh sweet cherries (about 12)** | 59 | 1 g | 14 g | 1 g | 2 g | 0 mg | 0 mg | 12 mg |
| **Meal Total** | 584 | 34 g | 93 g | 11.5 g (18%) | 14 g | 700 mg | 84 mg | 584 mg |

Grilled Red Snapper with Charred Tomato Salsa
White Rice (page 224)
Tarragon-Scented Broccoli and Cauliflower
Tossed Salad with Walnut Dressing
Fresh plums

# Grilled Red Snapper with Charred Tomato Salsa

*Total preparation time: 15 minutes*

Nonstick cooking spray
1¾ pounds red snapper fillet (substitute tuna, grouper, or other firm fish)
1 medium red onion, peeled and finely diced
4 medium green chiles, cored, seeded, and chopped
4 medium tomatoes, halved
2 tablespoons chopped fresh cilantro

1. Prepare grill and coat lightly with cooking spray.
2. Rinse fish and pat dry.
3. In a small bowl, combine onion and chiles. Mix well.
4. Place fish and tomatoes directly on grill over medium heat. Cook tomatoes 5 to 6 minutes, until just tender and slightly blackened; remove and set aside. Cook fish 8 to 10 minutes, or until fish flakes easily with a fork, turning once.
5. While fish is cooking, coarsely chop the tomato and add to onion mixture. Add cilantro and toss. Spoon mixture over fish and serve.

SERVES 4

# Tarragon–Scented Broccoli and Cauliflower

*Total preparation time: 12 minutes*

2 tablespoons chopped fresh tarragon *or* 2 teaspoons dried
1 pound broccoli, washed, tough ends removed, and cut into flowerets
1 pound cauliflower, washed, trimmed, and cut into flowerets
1 teaspoon olive oil

1. Fill a large saucepan with 2 inches water and set to boil.
2. Add chopped tarragon to water, and reduce heat to simmer. Place broccoli and cauliflower in a steaming basket or colander over water, and steam 5 minutes, or until crisp-tender. Toss with olive oil and serve.

SERVES 4

# Tossed Salad with Walnut Dressing

*Total preparation time: 10 minutes*

1 small head Boston or Bibb lettuce, outer leaves removed, washed, dried, and torn into bite-size pieces
1 small head iceberg lettuce, outer leaves removed, washed, dried, and torn into bite-size pieces
¼ cup chopped walnuts
¼ cup raspberry vinegar
2 teaspoons olive oil
2 cloves garlic, peeled and minced

1. Place greens and walnuts in a large salad bowl and toss.
2. In a small covered jar, combine vinegar, oil, and minced garlic. Shake well.
3. Dress immediately before serving.

SERVES 4

NUTRITIONAL INFORMATION PER SERVING

| | Calories | Protein | Carbohydrate | Fat | Fiber | Sodium | Cholesterol | Calcium |
|---|---|---|---|---|---|---|---|---|
| **Grilled Red Snapper with Charred Tomato Salsa** | 265 | 43 g | 15 g | 3 g | 3 g | 148 mg | 73 mg | 87 mg |
| **White Rice** | 105 | 29 g | 23 g | 0.4 g | 0.5 g | 0 mg | 0 mg | 3 mg |
| **Tossed Salad with Walnut Dressing** | 110 | 3 g | 10 g | 7 g | 3 g | 33 mg | 0 mg | 48 mg |
| **Tarragon-Scented Broccoli and Cauliflower** | 71 | 6 g | 12 g | 2 g | 6 g | 65 mg | 0 mg | 48 mg |
| **Fresh plums (2 medium)** | 72 | 1 g | 17 g | 1 g | 2 g | 0 mg | 0 mg | 5 mg |
| **Meal Total** | 623 | 55 g | 77 g | 13 g (19%) | 14.5 g | 246 mg | 73 mg | 143 mg |

**Herb–Rubbed Grilled Tuna**

**Corn on the Cob**

**Grilled Zucchini (page 220)**

**Steamed Green Beans (page 224)**

**Chopped Tomato-Cucumber Salad (page 192)**

**Raspberry sorbet**

# Herb-Rubbed Grilled Tuna

*Total preparation time: 30 minutes*

1 tablespoon chopped fresh basil

1 tablespoon chopped fresh mint

1 clove garlic, peeled and minced

1 tablespoon lemon juice

1 teaspoon olive oil

1¾ pounds fresh tuna fillet (substitute salmon, halibut, swordfish, or other firm fillet)

Nonstick cooking spray

1.   Place basil, mint, garlic, lemon juice, and olive oil in a food processor or blender and process until it forms a paste.
2.   Wash tuna and pat dry. Spread paste on the tuna, cover, and refrigerate 15 minutes.
3.   Prepare grill and coat lightly with cooking spray, or preheat broiler.
4.   Place tuna on grill or on a sheet under broiler and cook 5 minutes per side, until center of fish is translucent or internal temperature measures 145°.

SERVES 4

# Corn on the Cob

*Total preparation time: 8 minutes*

**4 small ears corn, husked (outer leaves and silk removed)**

1.   Fill large covered saucepan with 2 inches water and set to boil.
2.   Place corn in boiling water, cover, return to boil, then reduce heat to low. Simmer 5 to 6 minutes, or until tender. Do not overcook.

SERVES 4

NUTRITIONAL INFORMATION PER SERVING

|  | Calories | Protein | Carbohydrate | Fat | Fiber | Sodium | Cholesterol | Calcium |
|---|---|---|---|---|---|---|---|---|
| **Herb-Rubbed Tuna** | 217 | 44 g | 1 g | 3 g | 0 g | 74 mg | 93 mg | 61 mg |
| **Corn on the Cob** | 83 | 3 g | 19 g | 1 g | 2 g | 13 mg | 0 mg | 2 mg |
| **Grilled Zucchini** | 47 | 2 g | 11 g | 0 g | 2 g | 16 mg | 0 mg | 29 mg |
| **Steamed Green Beans** | 35 | 2 g | 8 g | 0 g | 4 g | 7 mg | 0 mg | 42 mg |
| **Tomato-Cucumber Salad** | 118 | 5 g | 19 g | 4 g | 6 g | 40 mg | 2 mg | 87 mg |
| **Raspberry sorbet (½ cup)** | 70 | 1 g | 17 g | 0 g | 0 g | 46 mg | 0 mg | 2 mg |
| **Meal Total** | 570 | 57 g | 75 g | 8 g (13%) | 14 g | 196 mg | 95 mg | 223 mg |

**Balsamic-Grilled Halibut Steak**
**Fennel-Onion Salad**
**Tomato Crostini**
**Steamed Spinach (page 163)**
**Mixed Berry Compote**

# Balsamic-Grilled Halibut Steak

*Total preparation time: 25 minutes*

**Nonstick cooking spray**
**½ cup fat-free balsamic vinaigrette dressing**
**1⅓ tablespoons lemon juice**
**4 cloves garlic, peeled and minced**
**Four 7-ounce halibut steaks, about ¾-inch thick**

1. Preheat broiler or prepare outdoor grill, and lightly coat broiler or grill rack with cooking spray.
2. In a shallow glass dish, combine the vinaigrette, lemon juice, and garlic. Add halibut steaks and turn to coat. Cover and marinate in refrigerator 15 minutes.
3. Grill or broil fish 4 to 6 inches from heat, turning once, about 7 minutes total, or until lightly translucent; cut fish in center to test for doneness.

SERVES 4

# Fennel–Onion Salad

*Total preparation time: 10 to 12 minutes*

¼ cup balsamic vinegar
1⅓ tablespoons granulated sugar
2 small heads red-leaf lettuce, outer leaves removed, washed, dried, and
   torn into bite-size pieces
4 cups fennel, tops and bottoms removed, washed, and thinly sliced
1 small red onion, peeled and thinly sliced

1.   In a small jar, combine vinegar and sugar. Shake well and set aside.
2.   In a large bowl, combine lettuce, sliced fennel, and sliced onion. Dress
     immediately before serving.

SERVES 4

# Tomato Crostini

*Total preparation time: 12 to 15 minutes*

½ loaf French bread, cut into eight 1-inch slices
2 large tomatoes, blanched, peeled, and chopped *or* 4 cups stewed tomatoes,
   well-drained
1⅓ tablespoons olive oil
1 tablespoon Italian seasoning or oregano

1.   Preheat broiler.
2.   Place bread on baking sheet and broil 1 to 2 minutes on each side until
     golden brown.
3.   Meanwhile, combine tomatoes, oil, and seasoning in a small bowl. Spread
     mixture onto each slice of toasted bread.

SERVES 4

# Mixed Berry Compote

*Total preparation time: 10 minutes*

1 pint strawberries, hulled, washed, and sliced
2 cups blueberries, rinsed
1 cup raspberries, rinsed
½ cup light whipped topping

Combine berries in a large mixing bowl and toss gently. Divide among 4 bowls, top each with 2 tablespoons whipped topping, and chill before serving.

SERVES 4

NUTRITIONAL INFORMATION PER SERVING

|  | Calories | Protein | Carbohydrate | Fat | Fiber | Sodium | Cholesterol | Calcium |
|---|---|---|---|---|---|---|---|---|
| **Balsamic-Grilled Halibut** | 244 | 42 g | 6 g | 5 g | 0 g | 115 mg | 64 mg | 108 mg |
| **Fennel-Onion Salad** | 74 | 3 g | 17 g | 0.5 g | 4 g | 54 mg | 0 mg | 79 mg |
| **Tomato Crostini** | 197 | 5 g | 30 g | 6 g | 3 g | 311 mg | 0 mg | 59 mg |
| **Steamed Spinach** | 36 | 5 g | 6 g | 0.5 g | 4 g | 129 mg | 0 mg | 162 mg |
| **Mixed Berry Compote** | 92 | 2 g | 27 g | 1.5 g | 10 g | 2 mg | 0 mg | 33 mg |
| **Meal Total** | 643 | 57 g | 86 g | 13.5 g (19%) | 21 g | 611 mg | 64 mg | 441 mg |

Lemon-Pepper Sole
Cinnamon-Dusted Sweet Potatoes
Steamed Spinach (page 163)
Oregano-Scented Summer Squash (page 163)
Tossed Salad with Tomatoes (page 159)
Fresh pear

## Lemon-Pepper Sole

*Total preparation time: 12 to 15 minutes*

Nonstick cooking spray
1¾ pounds skinless sole fillets, divided into 6- to 7-ounce portions
    (substitute flounder)
1 tablespoon olive oil
1 teaspoon lemon juice
½ teaspoon freshly ground black pepper
4 medium tomatoes, washed and sliced
2 medium scallions, trimmed and chopped
½ teaspoon dried basil

1. Preheat broiler, and spray rectangular baking dish with cooking spray.
2. Wash fish and pat dry. Brush fish with olive oil and lemon juice, then sprinkle with pepper. Place tomato slices on top of fish, and sprinkle with chopped scallion and basil.
3. Broil 5 to 7 minutes, or until fish flakes easily with fork.

SERVES 4

# Cinnamon–Dusted Sweet Potatoes

*Total preparation time: 10 to 15 or 60 to 70 minutes, depending on method*

**2 large sweet potatoes (or yams), with skin (see Note), scrubbed well, and ends trimmed**

**1 teaspoon ground cinnamon (substitute ground nutmeg, cloves, ginger, or allspice)**

*Oven method:* Preheat oven to 400°F. Prick potatoes a few times with a fork. Place on baking sheet and bake 50 to 60 minutes, or until soft when pierced by a fork. Allow to cool slightly before serving, 5 to 10 minutes. Split potatoes open and sprinkle with ground cinnamon, nutmeg, cloves, ginger, or allspice. *Microwave method:* Prick potatoes twice with a fork. Place side by side on a paper towel in center of microwave oven. Cook on high 5 to 8 minutes, or until soft when pierced by a fork. Sprinkle with ground cinnamon, nutmeg, cloves, ginger, or allspice.

Note: The skin of sweet potatoes contains many nutrients and fiber and should be left on and eaten whenever possible.

SERVES 4

NUTRITIONAL INFORMATION PER SERVING

|  | Calories | Protein | Carbohydrate | Fat | Fiber | Sodium | Cholesterol | Calcium |
|---|---|---|---|---|---|---|---|---|
| **Lemon-Pepper Sole** | 242 | 39 g | 7 g | 6 g | 2 g | 174 mg | 95 mg | 56 mg |
| **Cinnamon-Dusted Sweet Potatoes** | 99 | 2 g | 25 g | 0 g | 3 g | 34 mg | 0 mg | 22 mg |
| **Steamed Spinach** | 36 | 5 g | 6 g | 0.5 g | 4 g | 129 mg | 0 mg | 162 mg |
| **Oregano-Scented Summer Squash** | 23 | 1 g | 5 g | 0 g | 2 g | 2 mg | 0 mg | 27 mg |
| **Tossed Salad with Tomatoes** | 70 | 3 g | 15 g | 1 g | 4 g | 38 mg | 0 mg | 52 mg |
| **Fresh pear (1 medium)** | 98 | 1 g | 25 g | 1 g | 4 g | 0 mg | 0 mg | 18 mg |
| **Meal Total** | 568 | 51 g | 83 g | 8.1 g (13%) | 19 g | 377 mg | 95 mg | 337 mg |

# Vegetarian and Soy

White Bean and Tomato Salad

●

Tofu Vegetable Salad Platter

●

Stuffed Potato Olé

●

Polenta with Broiled Vegetables

●

Penne with Greens and White Beans

●

Spaghetti and Zucchini with Tofu Marinara

●

Vegetable Tofu Lasagna

●

Tempeh with Saucy Green Beans over White Rice

●

Veggie Tofu Stir-Fry with Sesame Seeds over Brown Rice

●

Baked Eggplant Parmesan

●

Quick Tortilla Pizza

●

Easy Bean Burrito

●

Vegetarian Chili

●

Savory Baked Soybeans

●

Tofu Cassoulet

●

**Low-fat cream of broccoli soup (ready-made)**
**White Bean and Tomato Salad**
**Whole wheat bread**
**Strawberry nonfat yogurt (artificially sweetened, ready-made)**

## White Bean and Tomato Salad

*Total preparation time: 75 minutes*

1 tablespoon white vinegar
1 tablespoon lemon juice
1 teaspoon Dijon mustard
1 drop liquid hot-pepper seasoning
2 teaspoons olive oil
One 16-ounce can small white beans, drained
½ tablespoon chopped fresh basil *or* 1 teaspoon dried
½ tablespoon chopped fresh mint *or* ½ teaspoon dried
1 tablespoon chopped fresh parsley
1 scallion, top and bottom removed, rinsed, and chopped
1 small clove garlic, peeled and minced
6 cherry tomatoes, washed and halved
½ large red bell pepper, washed, cored, seeded, and finely diced

1. In a small bowl, combine vinegar, lemon juice, mustard, and hot-pepper seasoning. Beating with a whisk or fork, slowly add the olive oil. Set aside.
2. In a large bowl, combine the drained beans with the basil, mint, parsley, scallion, and garlic. Mix in the dressing, cover, and refrigerate at least 15 minutes or up to 4 hours. Immediately before serving, lightly mix in tomatoes and bell peppers.

SERVES 4

NUTRITIONAL INFORMATION PER SERVING

| | Calories | Protein | Carbohydrate | Fat | Fiber | Sodium | Cholesterol | Calcium |
|---|---|---|---|---|---|---|---|---|
| White Bean and Tomato Salad | 166 | 9 g | 28 g | 3 g | 6 g | 189 mg | 0 mg | 94 mg |
| Low-fat cream of broccoli soup (1 cup) | 88 | 2 g | 13 g | 3 g | 2 g | 578 mg | 5 mg | 41 mg |
| Whole wheat bread (1 slice) | 69 | 3 g | 13 g | 1 g | 2 g | 148 mg | 0 mg | 20 mg |
| Strawberry nonfat yogurt (artificially sweetened, 1 cup) | 90 | 8 g | 14 g | 0 g | 2 g | 140 mg | 5 mg | 250 mg |
| Meal Total | 413 | 22 g | 68 g | 7 g (15%) | 12 g | 1,055 mg | 10 mg | 405 mg |

Barley soup (ready-made)
Tofu Vegetable Salad Platter
French roll
Honeydew wedge

# Tofu Vegetable Salad Platter

*Total preparation time: 35 minutes*

1 pound tofu, cut into ¼ x ¼ x 1-inch pieces
1 head Bibb lettuce, outer leaves removed, washed, dried, and leaves
  separated
2 large carrots, tops and bottoms removed, peeled, and grated
2 medium red peppers, cored, seeded, and cut into strips
2 stalks celery, washed and diced
2 cups alfalfa sprouts
2 large cucumbers, peeled and thinly sliced
½ medium red onion, peeled and thinly sliced

24 cherry tomatoes, washed and halved

2 ounces fat-free cheddar cheese, grated

¼ cup sunflower seeds

1 tablespoon olive oil

½ cup balsamic vinegar

1.  Preheat oven to 350°F.
2.  Place tofu in a colander and drain for 10 minutes. Pat dry with paper towels. Place on a baking sheet and bake at 350°F for 20 minutes. Remove and allow to cool.
3.  Lay lettuce leaves on large platter, and place baked tofu in center. Arrange grated carrots, pepper strips, diced celery, sprouts, sliced cucumbers, sliced onion, halved cherry tomatoes, and grated cheese around the tofu. Sprinkle sunflower seeds on top. Dress with oil and vinegar immediately before serving.

SERVES 4

NUTRITIONAL INFORMATION PER SERVING

|  | Calories | Protein | Carbohydrate | Fat | Fiber | Sodium | Cholesterol | Calcium |
|---|---|---|---|---|---|---|---|---|
| **Tofu Vegetable Salad Platter** | 265 | 18 g | 25 g | 13 g | 7 g | 265 mg | 0 mg | 275 mg |
| **Barley soup (1 cup)** | 90 | 6 g | 19 g | 0 g | 4 g | 210 mg | 0 mg | 40 mg |
| **French roll (1 ounce)** | 79 | 2 g | 14 g | 1 g | 1 g | 173 mg | 0 mg | 26 mg |
| **Honeydew wedge (⅛ melon)** | 56 | 1 g | 15 g | 0 g | 1 g | 16 mg | 0 mg | 10 mg |
| **Meal Total** | 490 | 27 g | 73 g | 14 g (20%) | 13 g | 664 mg | 0 mg | 351 mg |

Easy Minestrone Soup
Stuffed Potato Olé
Chopped Tomato–Cucumber Salad
Tangerines

## Easy Minestrone Soup

*Total preparation time: 20 minutes*

1 tablespoon olive oil
½ medium yellow onion, peeled and finely diced
1 clove garlic, peeled and minced
1 stalk celery, trimmed and finely diced
One 16-ounce can low-fat low-sodium vegetable broth
One 16-ounce can kidney beans
One 10-ounce package frozen mixed vegetables
1 medium Idaho potato, peeled, washed, and diced
¼ teaspoon dried basil
⅛ teaspoon ground black pepper

1.  Heat oil in a medium Dutch oven over medium heat. Add onions, garlic, and celery and sauté 3 to 4 minutes, until onion is wilted and golden.
2.  Add broth, beans, vegetables, potatoes, basil, and pepper. Bring to a boil, then reduce heat to low and simmer 15 minutes. Serve warm.

SERVES 4

# Stuffed Potato Olé

*Total preparation time: 15 minutes or 60 to 70 minutes, depending on method*

**4 medium baking potatoes, well-scrubbed**
**½ pound reduced-fat sharp cheddar cheese, shredded**
**1 red pepper, washed, cored, seeded, and finely diced**
**4 tablespoons chopped chives**
**4 tablespoons nonfat sour cream**

1.　Bake potato. *Oven method:* Preheat oven to 400°F. Prick each potato a few times with a fork, place on baking sheet, and cook 50 to 60 minutes, or until soft when pricked by a fork. *Microwave method:* Prick each potato a few times with a fork, place side by side on a paper towel in center of microwave oven, and cook on high 5 to 8 minutes, or until soft when pricked by a fork.
2.　Preheat broiler. Split baked potatoes and top with shredded cheese. Place potatoes on a tray and broil until cheese begins to melt, 4 to 5 minutes. Remove from broiler and top with diced pepper, chopped chives, and sour cream.

SERVES 4

# Chopped Tomato–Cucumber Salad

*Total preparation time: 10 minutes*

1 small head iceberg lettuce, outer leaves removed, washed, dried, and torn
    into bite-size pieces
1 small head red-leaf lettuce, outer leaves removed, washed, dried, and torn
    into bite-size pieces
4 large cucumbers, peeled and thinly sliced
4 medium tomatoes, washed and quartered
½ cup fat-free dressing

Place greens in a large salad bowl and toss with cucumbers and tomatoes.
Dress immediately before serving.

SERVES 4

NUTRITIONAL INFORMATION PER SERVING

|  | Calories | Protein | Carbohydrate | Fat | Fiber | Sodium | Cholesterol | Calcium |
|---|---|---|---|---|---|---|---|---|
| **Easy Minestrone Soup** | 224 | 10 g | 37 g | 5 g | 8 g | 483 mg | 2 mg | 68 mg |
| **Stuffed Potato Olé** | 313 | 22 g | 36 g | 9 g | 3 g | 218 mg | 30 mg | 550 mg |
| **Tomato-Cucumber Salad** | 118 | 5 g | 19 g | 4 g | 6 g | 40 mg | 2 mg | 87 mg |
| **Tangerines (2 small)** | 74 | 1 g | 19 g | 0 g | 4 g | 2 mg | 0 mg | 24 mg |
| **Meal Total** | 729 | 38 g | 111 g | 18 g (22%) | 21 g | 743 mg | 34 mg | 729 mg |

Tomato juice cocktail with lemon wedge (ready-made)
Polenta with Broiled Vegetables
Tossed Salad with Sprouts, Seeds, and Beans
Frozen nonfat yogurt

## Polenta with Broiled Vegetables

*Total preparation time: 25 minutes*

1 cup polenta (ground cornmeal)
4 teaspoons olive oil
¼ cup balsamic vinegar
4 tablespoons chopped fresh basil
4 cloves garlic, minced
¼ teaspoon ground pepper
2 yellow peppers, washed, cored, seeded, and sliced
4 medium onions, peeled and quartered
4 tomatoes, washed and quartered
6 large mushrooms, washed and halved

1. Preheat broiler.
2. In a large bowl, combine cornmeal with 1 cup cold water. Stir to mix. Set 3 more cups water to boil in a medium saucepan over medium heat. When water begins to boil, *gradually* stir in cornmeal mixture. Reduce heat immediately to low, cover, and steam 15 minutes, stirring frequently.
3. Meanwhile, combine olive oil, vinegar, basil, garlic, and pepper in a large mixing bowl. Add the vegetables and toss well to coat.
4. Place vegetables on a cookie sheet or broiling pan. Broil under high heat until al dente, about 8 to 10 minutes. Do not overcook.
5. Top cooked polenta with vegetables and serve.

SERVES 4

# Tossed Salad with Sprouts, Seeds, and Beans

*Total preparation time: 10 minutes*

1 head Boston or Bibb lettuce, outer leaves removed, washed, dried, and
   torn into bite-size pieces
1 small head iceberg lettuce, outer leaves removed, washed, dried, and torn
   into bite-size pieces
24 cherry tomatoes, washed and halved
1 cup alfalfa sprouts
One 15-ounce can kidney beans, drained
½ cup fat-free salad dressing
4 tablespoons sunflower seeds

In a large salad bowl, toss lettuce with tomatoes, sprouts, and kidney
beans. Immediately before serving, dress, divide evenly among 4 salad
plates, and top each with 1 tablespoon sunflower seeds.

SERVES 4

NUTRITIONAL INFORMATION PER SERVING

|  | Calories | Protein | Carbohydrate | Fat | Fiber | Sodium | Cholesterol | Calcium |
|---|---|---|---|---|---|---|---|---|
| Tomato juice cocktail with lemon wedge (1 cup) | 60 | 2 g | 11 g | 0 g | 2 g | 140 mg | 0 mg | 40 mg |
| Polenta | 190 | 5 g | 39 g | 1 g | 2 g | 1 mg | 0 mg | 2 mg |
| Broiled Vegetables | 137 | 4 g | 21 g | 5.5 g | 4 g | 20 mg | 0 mg | 44 mg |
| Tossed Salad with Sprouts, Seeds, and Beans | 201 | 11 g | 31 g | 5 g | 8 g | 404 mg | 0 mg | 102 mg |
| Frozen nonfat yogurt (½ cup) | 95 | 5 g | 19 g | 0 g | 0 g | 64 mg | 2 mg | 167 mg |
| Meal Total | 683 | 27 g | 121 g | 11.5 g (15%) | 16 g | 629 mg | 2 mg | 355 mg |

Penne with Greens and White Beans
Asparagus Spears (page 226)
Tomato, Egg, and Cucumber Salad
Strawberries

## Penne with Greens and White Beans

*Total preparation time: 25 minutes*

4 teaspoons olive oil
4 cloves garlic, peeled and minced
1 medium red bell pepper, washed, cored, seeded, and diced
2 pounds fresh greens (spinach, kale, Swiss chard, or escarole), washed
   thoroughly (but not dried), stems removed, and torn into bite-size pieces
4 teaspoons balsamic vinegar
¼ cup vegetable stock
Two 15-ounce cans cannellini or other white beans, drained
8 ounces penne (substitute other tubular pasta such as rotini or ziti)
¼ cup grated Parmesan cheese

1. Set a large covered pot to boil for pasta.
2. Heat the oil in a large nonstick skillet over medium-high heat. Add garlic and pepper, and sauté 2 minutes. Stir in greens, vinegar, and stock, cover pan, and cook until greens are wilted and tender but still bright green, 5 to 7 minutes. Gently stir the beans into greens mixture, set aside, and keep warm until pasta is ready.
3. Meanwhile, cook pasta according to package directions, until al dente. Drain.
4. Add pasta to greens-beans mixture and gently mix. Top each serving with 1 tablespoon grated Parmesan.

SERVES 4

# Tomato, Egg, and Cucumber Salad

*Total preparation time: 15 minutes*

4 large eggs
½ cup balsamic vinegar
4 teaspoons olive oil
4 medium tomatoes, washed and cut into ¼-inch slices
2 large cucumbers, peeled and thinly sliced
½ head red- or green-leaf lettuce, outer leaves removed, washed, dried, and
    separated into leaves

1.  Place eggs in a saucepan with water to cover at least 1 inch above eggs,
    and bring to a boil. Immediately after water has boiled, reduce heat to just
    below simmering, cover, and cook eggs 15 to 20 minutes. Cool at once in
    cold water (this prevents the yolk from darkening and makes for easier
    peeling). Once cool, peel and slice into ¼-inch slices.
2.  Meanwhile, combine vinegar and oil in small covered jar; shake well.
3.  Toss tomatoes, cucumbers, and lettuce in a large salad bowl. Immediately
    before serving, toss with dressing, and top with sliced egg.

SERVES 4

NUTRITIONAL INFORMATION PER SERVING

|  | Calories | Protein | Carbohydrate | Fat | Fiber | Sodium | Cholesterol | Calcium |
|---|---|---|---|---|---|---|---|---|
| Penne with Greens and White Beans | 520 | 26 g | 85 g | 9 g | 14 g | 839 mg | 5 mg | 409 mg |
| Asparagus Spears | 39 | 4 g | 8 g | 0.5 g | 3.5 g | 3 mg | 0 mg | 36 mg |
| Tomato, Egg, and Cucumber Salad | 190 | 9 g | 16 g | 11 g | 3 g | 90 mg | 212 mg | 73 mg |
| Strawberries | 50 | 1 g | 12 g | 0.6 g | 4 g | 2 mg | 0 mg | 23 mg |
| Meal Total | 799 | 40 g | 121 g | 21.1 g (24%) | 24.5 g | 934 mg | 217 mg | 541 mg |

Spaghetti and Zucchini with Tofu Marinara
Mixed Green Salad
Fat-free pudding

# Spaghetti and Zucchini with Tofu Marinara

*Total preparation time: 80 minutes*

1 pound firm tofu
8 ounces spaghetti
1 tablespoon olive oil
1 medium onion, peeled and thinly sliced
4 cloves garlic, peeled and minced
2 medium zucchini, scrubbed, tops and bottoms removed, and cut into
    ¼-inch slices
4 medium tomatoes, washed and diced
One 8-ounce can tomato sauce
1 bay leaf
¼ teaspoon ground black pepper
¼ teaspoon dried basil
¼ teaspoon dried oregano
¼ cup grated Parmesan cheese

1. Break tofu into coarse chunks and drain in a colander 10 minutes. Wrap in paper towels for 20 minutes.
2. Meanwhile, set a large pot of water to boil. Cook spaghetti according to package directions until al dente, 10 to 12 minutes. Remove from heat, drain, set aside in a large serving bowl, and keep warm.
3. Meanwhile, spread oil in a large nonstick pan and set over medium-high heat. Add onion and garlic and sauté until onions are translucent, 3 to 4

minutes. Add zucchini and tofu and sauté 5 to 10 minutes until tofu browns. Add tomatoes, tomato sauce, bay leaf, pepper, basil, and oregano and reduce heat to low. Cover and simmer 15 minutes. Uncover and simmer an additional 10 minutes. Remove and discard bay leaf.

4. Pour the cooked sauce over the cooked spaghetti, and top with grated Parmesan.

SERVES 4

# Mixed Green Salad

*Total preparation time: 10 minutes*

1 small head red- or green-leaf lettuce, outer leaves removed, washed, dried, and torn into bite-size pieces
1 small head romaine lettuce, outer leaves removed, washed, dried, and torn into bite-size pieces
1 dozen button mushrooms, washed, dried, and thinly sliced
2 medium sweet red peppers, washed, cored, seeded, and diced
4 medium tomatoes, washed and quartered
½ cup fat-free salad dressing

Toss all ingredients except dressing in large salad bowl. Dress immediately before serving.

SERVES 4

NUTRITIONAL INFORMATION PER SERVING

|  | Calories | Protein | Carbohydrate | Fat | Fiber | Sodium | Cholesterol | Calcium |
|---|---|---|---|---|---|---|---|---|
| Spaghetti and Zucchini with Tofu Marinara | 381 | 20 g | 55 g | 11 g | 9 g | 167 mg | 5 mg | 297 mg |
| Mixed Green Salad | 115 | 6 g | 24 g | 1 g | 7 g | 44 mg | 0 mg | 131 mg |
| Fat-free pudding (4 ounces) | 100 | 2 g | 23 g | 0 g | 0 g | 241 mg | 0 mg | 80 mg |
| Meal Total | 596 | 28 g | 102 g | 12 g (18%) | 16 g | 452 mg | 5 mg | 508 mg |

Vegetable Tofu Lasagna
Tossed Salad (page 162)
Italian bread
Diet gelatin with sliced kiwi

## Vegetable Tofu Lasagna

*Total preparation time: 2 hours*

1 pound firm tofu
8 ounces dry lasagna noodles
1 tablespoon olive oil
3 cloves garlic, peeled and minced
½ small yellow onion, peeled and finely diced
1 pound button mushrooms, washed, dried, and thinly sliced
1 teaspoon dried basil
1 teaspoon dried oregano
Two 15-ounce cans tomato sauce
One 6-ounce can tomato paste
1 pound fresh spinach, ends removed, well washed, dried, and chopped
1 pound carrots, tops and bottoms removed, peeled, and grated
1 pound zucchini, tops and bottoms removed, scrubbed, and grated
½ pound part-skim ricotta cheese
¼ cup soy Parmesan cheese, grated

1. Preheat oven to 400°F, and bring 3 quarts water to boil in a large stockpot.
2. Break tofu into coarse chunks and drain in a colander 10 minutes. Remove and wrap in paper towels for 20 minutes to remove excess moisture. Set aside.

3. Add lasagna noodles to boiling water, and cook according to package directions until al dente; do not overcook. Drain, set aside, and keep warm.

4. Meanwhile, heat oil over medium-high heat in a large skillet or Dutch oven. Add drained tofu, minced garlic, diced onions, sliced mushrooms, basil, and oregano. Cook, stirring often, until onions are soft and liquid has evaporated, 6 to 7 minutes. Add tomato sauce and tomato paste and stir to blend; set aside.

5. In a large bowl, mix chopped spinach, grated carrots, and grated zucchini with ricotta cheese.

6. Assemble the lasagna in a 9 x 13-inch baking dish: spread a third of the tomato sauce on bottom of pan and arrange half the noodles, overlapping slightly, on top of the sauce. Spread half of the vegetable-ricotta mixture on top of the noodles. Repeat with another layer of sauce, noodles, and vegetable-ricotta. Top with the remaining sauce and sprinkle with the grated Parmesan.

7. Bake, uncovered, at 400°F until hot in the center, 25 to 30 minutes. Let stand 10 minutes before serving.

SERVES 6

NUTRITIONAL INFORMATION PER SERVING

|  | Calories | Protein | Carbohydrate | Fat | Fiber | Sodium | Cholesterol | Calcium |
|---|---|---|---|---|---|---|---|---|
| **Vegetable Tofu Lasagna** | 457 | 27 g | 62 g | 14 g | 10 g | 306 mg | 26 mg | 511 mg |
| **Tossed Salad** | 88 | 5 g | 18 g | 1 g | 5 g | 35 mg | 0 mg | 73 mg |
| **Italian bread** | 77 | 2.5 g | 14 g | 1 g | 1 g | 165 mg | 0 mg | 22 mg |
| **Diet gelatin (1 cup) with sliced kiwi (1)** | 70 | 5 g | 14 g | 0.5 g | 2 g | 0 mg | 0 mg | 30 mg |
| **Meal Total** | 692 | 39.5 g | 108 g | 16.5 g (21%) | 18 g | 506 mg | 26 mg | 636 mg |

Tempeh with Saucy Green Beans over Rice
Five–Veggie Salad
Banana

# Tempeh with Saucy Green Beans over Rice

*Total preparation time: 55 minutes*

1 cup uncooked white rice
Two 8-ounce cakes tempeh
3 tablespoons tamari
1 tablespoon sesame oil
½ medium yellow onion, peeled and finely diced
3 large cloves garlic, peeled and minced
1 red chili pepper, washed, cored, seeded, and finely diced
One 8-ounce can tomato sauce
4 ounces tomato paste
1 pound green beans, stringed, trimmed, and washed

1.  Place rice and 2 cups water in medium saucepan. Cover and bring to a boil. Reduce heat to low and simmer for 15 to 20 minutes, or until all the water is absorbed.
2.  Cut tempeh in half widthwise, then cut into strips (similar to bacon). Place in a shallow dish with tamari, cover, and refrigerate 15 minutes, turning once.
3.  Meanwhile, add oil to a wok or large nonstick skillet and heat over medium-high flame. Add onion, garlic, and chili pepper and stir-fry until onions wilt, 1 to 2 minutes. Drain tempeh, add to wok, and stir-fry 5 to 7 minutes, until golden brown. Add tomato sauce, tomato paste, and green beans, bring to a near-boil, then immediately reduce heat to low, cover, and simmer 10 minutes. Serve immediately over the cooked white rice.

SERVES 4

# Five-Veggie Salad

*Total preparation time: 10 minutes*

2 large tomatoes, washed, quartered, and thinly sliced

1 large cucumber, peeled and thinly sliced

2 stalks celery, trimmed and diced

2 large carrots, tops and bottoms removed, peeled and shredded

6 radishes, trimmed and sliced

1 tablespoon chopped parsley

2 tablespoons lemon juice

1 tablespoon olive oil

1 clove garlic, peeled and minced

1. In a large bowl, toss tomatoes, cucumber, celery, carrots, radishes, and parsley.
2. In a small covered jar, combine lemon juice, olive oil, and garlic. Shake well.
3. Dress salad immediately before serving.

SERVES 4

NUTRITIONAL INFORMATION PER SERVING

|  | Calories | Protein | Carbohydrate | Fat | Fiber | Sodium | Cholesterol | Calcium |
|---|---|---|---|---|---|---|---|---|
| **Tempeh with Saucy Green Beans over Rice** | 531 | 31 g | 80 g | 13 g | 13.5 g | 809 mg | 0 mg | 194 mg |
| **Five-Veggie Salad** | 82 | 2 g | 12 g | 3 g | 3 g | 42 mg | 0 mg | 37 mg |
| **Banana (1 medium)** | 109 | 1 g | 28 g | 1 g | 3 g | 1 mg | 0 mg | 7 mg |
| **Meal Total** | 722 | 34 g | 120 g | 16.6 g (21%) | 19.5 g | 852 mg | 0 mg | 238 mg |

Tomato soup (ready-made; see page 149)
Easy Veggie Tofu Stir-Fry with Sesame Seeds over Brown Rice
Berry-Peach Salad

## Easy Veggie Tofu Stir-Fry with Sesame Seeds over Brown Rice

*Total preparation time: 1 hour*

2 pounds firm tofu, cut into 1-inch cubes

3 tablespoons light (reduced-sodium) soy sauce

2¼ cups vegetable broth or water

¾ cup brown rice

1 tablespoon canola or olive oil

4 cloves garlic, peeled and minced

1 medium yellow onion, peeled and thinly sliced

1 pound broccoli, washed, trimmed, and cut into bite-size pieces

2 large red peppers, washed, cored, seeded, and thinly sliced

½ pound button mushrooms, washed and thinly sliced

One 6-ounce can water chestnuts, drained

½ teaspoon dried basil

½ teaspoon dried oregano

½ teaspoon ground black pepper

¼ cup sesame seeds

1. Place tofu in a colander and drain 10 minutes. Pat dry with paper towels. Place soy sauce in a shallow dish, add tofu, cover, refrigerate, and marinate 15 minutes, or up to 1 hour, turning once.

2. In medium covered saucepan, bring 2 cups vegetable broth or water to a boil. Slowly stir in rice, cover, and reduce heat to low. Simmer 40 minutes, or until all the water is absorbed.

3.  Meanwhile, heat the oil in a wok, large skillet, or heavy saucepan over medium-high flame. Add garlic and onion and sauté until onions are wilted, 1 to 2 minutes. Add broccoli and red peppers, the remaining ¼ cup broth or water, and cook, stirring frequently, 5 minutes. Add mushrooms, water chestnuts, basil, oregano, and black pepper and continue to cook 2 more minutes, or until mushrooms are soft. Add sesame seeds and the marinated tofu with soy sauce, and cook, stirring gently, until tofu is heated through, about 5 minutes. Serve over the cooked rice.

SERVES 4

# Berry–Peach Salad

*Total preparation time: 10 minutes*

1 pint strawberries, hulled, washed, sliced
1 pint blueberries, washed, cleaned
4 medium peaches, washed, pitted, sliced
½ teaspoon lemon juice
1 packet sugar substitute (optional)

In large bowl, combine strawberries, blueberries, and peaches with lemon juice. Sprinkle with sugar substitute, if desired. Serve chilled.

SERVES 4

NUTRITIONAL INFORMATION PER SERVING

|  | Calories | Protein | Carbohydrate | Fat | Fiber | Sodium | Cholesterol | Calcium |
|---|---|---|---|---|---|---|---|---|
| Tomato soup (1 cup) | 99 | 3 g | 19 g | 1 g | 4 g | 480 mg | 0 mg | 56 mg |
| Easy Veggie Tofu Stir-Fry with Sesame Seeds over Brown Rice | 387 | 20 g | 51 g | 14 g | 8 g | 463 mg | 0 mg | 289 mg |
| Berry-Peach Salad | 102 | 2 g | 29 g | 0.5 g | 7 g | 39 mg | 0 mg | 24 mg |
| Meal Total | 588 | 25 g | 99 g | 15.5 g | 19 g | 982 mg | 0 mg | 369 mg |

Baked Eggplant Parmesan
Multicolored Salad (page 218)
Fruit salad (ready–made)

# Baked Eggplant Parmesan

*Total preparation time: 85 minutes*

Nonstick cooking spray
¾ cup soy milk or skim milk
1 cup bread crumbs
1 cup wheat germ
1 teaspoon basil
½ teaspoon oregano
½ teaspoon thyme
¼ teaspoon salt
2 medium eggplants, washed, ends removed, and cut into ½-inch slices
2 cups tomato sauce
½ pound fat-free mozzarella cheese
½ cup grated Parmesan cheese

1. Preheat oven to 375°F. Spray nonstick baking sheet with cooking spray.
2. Place milk in shallow bowl.
3. In second bowl, combine bread crumbs, wheat germ, basil, oregano, thyme, and salt.
4. Dip eggplant slices first in milk, then dip in bread crumb mixture to coat both sides. Place prepared eggplant on baking sheet. Bake at 375°F until tender, about 25 to 30 minutes. Remove from oven, cover, and keep warm.

5.   In large casserole dish, spread ¼ cup tomato sauce on bottom of pan. Add a layer of eggplant, then tomato sauce, then mozzarella cheese. Repeat layers until ingredients are used. Sprinkle top with Parmesan cheese.

6.   Bake, uncovered, at 375°F for 45 minutes, or until edges are bubbly. Let sit for 10 minutes before cutting. Serve hot.

SERVES 4

NUTRITIONAL INFORMATION PER SERVING

|  | Calories | Protein | Carbohydrate | Fat | Fiber | Sodium | Cholesterol | Calcium |
|---|---|---|---|---|---|---|---|---|
| **Baked Eggplant Parmesan** | 483 | 39 g | 63 g | 10 g | 14 g | 1,085 mg | 20 mg | 1,109 mg |
| **Multicolored Salad** | 85 | 3 g | 18 g | 1 g | 3 g | 78 mg | 0 mg | 127 mg |
| **Fruit salad (1 cup)** | 74 | 1 g | 19 g | 0 g | 2 g | 7 mg | 0 mg | 17 mg |
| **Meal Total** | 642 | 43 g | 100 g | 11 g (15%) | 19 g | 1,170 mg | 20 mg | 1,253 mg |

Quick Tortilla Pizza
Avocado Salad
Cucumber spears
Fresh sliced strawberries

# Quick Tortilla Pizza

*Total preparation time: 15 to 25 minutes*

**4 large flour tortillas (see Note)**
**One 16-ounce can fat-free refried beans**
**2 large tomatoes, washed and chopped**
**½ cup shredded reduced-fat sharp cheese**
**½ head iceberg lettuce, outer leaves removed, washed, dried, and shredded**
**2 cups salsa**
**12 large ripe pitted black olives, very thinly sliced**
**¼ cup nonfat sour cream**

1.  Preheat broiler.
2.  Place tortillas on a baking sheet. Layer beans, tomatoes, and cheese evenly among tortillas and broil 2 to 3 minutes, or until cheese melts.
3.  Remove from oven and top each with equal portions of the shredded lettuce, salsa, sliced olives, and sour cream.

SERVES 4

Note: To warm tortillas in the microwave, place flat in microwave and heat on medium 45 to 50 seconds until hot; do not overheat. *Oven method:* Wrap tortillas in aluminum foil and warm in 250°F oven 10 minutes.

# Avocado Salad

*Total preparation time: 10 to 12 minutes*

1 small head iceberg lettuce, outer leaves removed, washed, dried, and torn
   into bite-size pieces
1 small head red-leaf lettuce, outer leaves removed, washed, dried, and torn
   into bite-size pieces
1 medium ripe avocado, peeled, pitted, and diced
1 small red onion, peeled and thinly sliced
½ cup balsamic vinegar

Place lettuce in a large bowl and toss with diced avocado and sliced
onion. Dress with balsamic vinegar immediately before serving.

SERVES 4

## NUTRITIONAL INFORMATION PER SERVING

|  | Calories | Protein | Carbohydrate | Fat | Fiber | Sodium | Cholesterol | Calcium |
|---|---|---|---|---|---|---|---|---|
| Quick Tortilla Pizza | 395 | 19 g | 63 g | 8 g | 11 g | 1,432 mg | 8 mg | 289 mg |
| Avocado Salad | 127 | 3 g | 13 g | 8 g | 5 g | 27 mg | 0 mg | 56 mg |
| Cucumber spears | 12 | 0.5 g | 3 g | 0 g | 0.7 g | 2 mg | 0 mg | 14 mg |
| Fresh sliced strawberries (1 cup) | 50 | 1 g | 12 g | 0.6 g | 4 g | 2 mg | 0 mg | 23 mg |
| Meal Total | 584 | 23.5 g | 91 g | 16.6 g (26%) | 20.7 g | 1,463 mg | 8 mg | 382 mg |

**Gazpacho (ready–made)**
**Easy Bean Burrito**
**Fat-free tortilla chips**
**Mandarin oranges**

## Easy Bean Burrito

*Total preparation time: 15 to 25 minutes*

1 tablespoon olive oil
4 cloves garlic, peeled and minced
½ medium yellow onion, peeled and diced
One 16-ounce can black beans, drained
One 16-ounce can corn kernels, drained
4 medium flour tortillas, warmed (see Note)
¼ pound reduced-fat Monterey Jack cheese, shredded
½ head iceberg lettuce, outer leaves removed, washed, dried, and shredded
1 scallion, top and bottom removed, washed and chopped
¼ cup nonfat sour cream

1.  Heat oil in a large nonstick skillet over medium-high flame. Add garlic and onion and sauté until golden, 4 minutes. Add beans and corn, reduce heat to low, and cook until mixture is heated through, 4 to 5 minutes.
2.  Lay tortillas on a work surface. Evenly divide the bean mixture among the tortillas, and top with the shredded cheese, shredded lettuce, and chopped scallions. Roll the tortillas, and top each with 1 tablespoon sour cream.

SERVES 4

Note: To warm tortillas in the microwave, place flat in microwave and heat on medium 45 to 50 seconds until hot; do not overheat. *Oven method:* Wrap tortillas in aluminum foil and warm in 250°F oven 10 minutes.

NUTRITIONAL INFORMATION PER SERVING

|  | Calories | Protein | Carbohydrate | Fat | Fiber | Sodium | Cholesterol | Calcium |
|---|---|---|---|---|---|---|---|---|
| Gazpacho (1 cup) | 46 | 7 g | 4 g | 0.5 g | 0.5 g | 739 mg | 0 mg | 24 mg |
| Easy Bean Burrito | 552 | 28 g | 84 g | 13.5 g | 16 g | 439 mg | 15 mg | 386 mg |
| 10 Fat-free tortilla chips | 61 | 2 g | 12 g | 1 g | 1 g | 89 mg | 0 mg | 33 mg |
| Mandarin oranges (½ cup) | 53 | 1 g | 12 g | 0 g | 0 g | 0 mg | 0 mg | 15 mg |
| Meal Total | 712 | 38 g | 112 g | 15 g (19%) | 17.5 g | 1,267 mg | 15 mg | 458 mg |

Vegetarian Chili with Rice
Mixed Green Salad (page 198)
Cantaloupe wedge

## Vegetarian Chili with Rice

*Total preparation time: 60 minutes*

3/4 cup brown rice
1 tablespoon olive oil
4 small cloves garlic, peeled and minced
1 medium yellow onion, peeled and finely diced
2 celery stalks, washed, trimmed, and finely diced
2 large carrots, trimmed, washed, and diced
One 32-ounce can stewed tomatoes in juice
One 16-ounce can garbanzo beans, drained
3 cups canned kidney beans, drained (1 large 24-ounce can)
2 teaspoons chili powder
1/2 teaspoon ground black pepper
1/2 cup shredded reduced-fat sharp cheese

1. Bring 2 cups water to a boil in a medium covered saucepan. Slowly stir in rice, cover, reduce heat to low, and simmer 40 minutes, or until all the water is absorbed.
2. Meanwhile, heat oil in a Dutch oven or large covered heavy saucepan over medium-high flame. Add garlic and sauté until golden, about 30 seconds. Add onions, celery, and carrots and sauté, stirring frequently, until onions are soft, 3 to 4 minutes. Stir in tomatoes, garbanzos, kidney beans,

chili powder, and black pepper. Increase heat to high and bring to a boil, then reduce heat to low, cover, and simmer 10 minutes.

3. Serve over the cooked brown rice, and top each serving with 2 tablespoons shredded cheese.

SERVES 4

NUTRITIONAL INFORMATION PER SERVING

|  | Calories | Protein | Carbohydrate | Fat | Fiber | Sodium | Cholesterol | Calcium |
|---|---|---|---|---|---|---|---|---|
| **Vegetarian Chili with Rice** | 575 | 26 g | 104 g | 7 g | 19 g | 1,200 mg | 3 mg | 434 mg |
| **Mixed Green Salad** | 115 | 6 g | 24 g | 1 g | 7 g | 44 mg | 0 mg | 131 mg |
| **Cantaloupe wedge (1/8 melon)** | 24 | 1 g | 6 g | 0.5 g | 0.5 g | 6 mg | 0 mg | 8 mg |
| **Meal Total** | 714 | 33 g | 134 g | 8.5 g (10%) | 26.5 g | 1,250 mg | 3 mg | 573 mg |

Savory Baked Soybeans
Tomato, Egg, and Cucumber Salad (page 196)
Mixed Berry Compote (page 183)

# Savory Baked Soybeans

*Total preparation time: 3 to 4 hours to prepare soybeans; 3 hours to prepare casserole*

2 cups cooked soybeans, drained

2 cups tomato sauce

1 large yellow onion, peeled and finely diced

2 cloves garlic, peeled and minced

1 teaspoon dry mustard

2 teaspoons chili powder

¼ teaspoon ground black pepper

2 tablespoons dark molasses

1.  Preheat oven to 300°F.
2.  In a large Dutch oven or ovenproof pot, combine 2 quarts of water with all ingredients. Bake in 300°F oven 3 hours, stirring occasionally. If casserole becomes dry during cooking, add water in small increments. Allow to cool 10 minutes before serving.

SERVES 4

NUTRITIONAL INFORMATION PER SERVING

|  | Calories | Protein | Carbohydrate | Fat | Fiber | Sodium | Cholesterol | Calcium |
|---|---|---|---|---|---|---|---|---|
| Savory Baked Soybeans | 451 | 35 g | 43 g | 19 g | 11 g | 173 mg | 0 mg | 330 mg |
| Tomato, Egg, and Cucumber Salad | 190 | 9 g | 16 g | 11 g | 3 g | 90 mg | 212 mg | 73 mg |
| Mixed Berry Compote | 88 | 1 g | 23 g | 1.5 g | 7 g | 2 mg | 0 mg | 26 mg |
| Meal Total | 733 | 46 g | 86 g | 31.5 g (39%) | 24 g | 265 mg | 212 mg | 436 mg |

Tofu Cassoulet
Mushroom Bouillon (page 321)
Wild Rice (page 169)
Asparagus Spears (page 226)
Fresh plums

## Tofu Cassoulet

*Total preparation time: 70 minutes*

1 pound firm tofu, cut into 1-inch cubes
Nonstick cooking spray
1 tablespoon olive oil
4 cloves garlic, peeled and minced
2 medium carrots, tops and bottoms removed, peeled and shredded
½ medium yellow onion, peeled and finely diced
2 medium tomatoes, washed and chopped
½ pound button mushrooms, washed, dried, and sliced
1 pound fresh spinach, ends removed, well washed and dried
¼ teaspoon dried oregano
¼ teaspoon dried basil
¼ teaspoon ground black pepper
One 16-ounce can white beans (navy or cannellini), drained
¾ cup salsa
4 ounces fat-free or soy mozzarella cheese, shredded

1. Preheat oven to 350°F.
2. Place tofu in a colander and drain for 20 minutes. Pat dry with paper towels, crumble into small pieces, and set aside.
3. Spray a large nonstick skillet with vegetable cooking spray. Add half the oil and sauté tofu over medium-high heat until browned, 5 to 10 minutes. Remove from pan and set aside.

4.   Add garlic, carrots, onion, and remaining oil to pan and sauté until onion is translucent, 3 to 4 minutes. Add tomatoes and cook until soft, another 3 to 4 minutes. Add mushrooms and spinach, and continue cooking until spinach is wilted but still bright green, 2 minutes. Add oregano, basil, and pepper. Mix gently and remove from heat.

5.   In a large Dutch oven or baking dish, layer half the beans, top with half the cooked vegetables, half the salsa, half the tofu, and half the mozzarella. Repeat the layers with the other half of the ingredients, ending with cheese on top.

6.   Bake in 350°F oven 35 minutes, or until cheese is lightly golden. Allow to cool 10 minutes before serving.

SERVES 4

NUTRITIONAL INFORMATION PER SERVING

|  | Calories | Protein | Carbohydrate | Fat | Fiber | Sodium | Cholesterol | Calcium |
|---|---|---|---|---|---|---|---|---|
| **Tofu Cassoulet** | 390 | 28 g | 46 g | 13 g | 12 g | 589 mg | 16 mg | 520 mg |
| **Mushroom Bouillon** | 48 | 4 g | 4.5 g | 1 g | 1 g | 59 mg | 0 mg | 17 mg |
| **Wild Rice** | 80 | 3 g | 17 g | 0 g | 1 g | 2 mg | 0 mg | 2 mg |
| **Asparagus Spears** | 39 | 4 g | 8 g | 0.5 g | 3.5 g | 3 mg | 0 mg | 36 mg |
| **Plums (2 medium)** | 73 | 1 g | 17 g | 1 g | 2 g | 0 mg | 0 mg | 5 mg |
| **Meal Total** | 630 | 40 g | 92.5 g | 15.5 g (22%) | 19.5 g | 653 mg | 16 mg | 580 mg |

# Beef and Lamb

**Grilled Sirloin**

●

**Cajun Grilled Flank Steak**

●

**Veal Chops with Papaya Salsa**

●

**Greek-Style Burrito**

●

**Mint-Glazed Lamb Chop**

---

**Grilled Sirloin**
**Garlicky Oven Fries**
**Asparagus Spears (page 226)**
**Parsley Carrot Coins (page 163)**
**Multicolored Salad**
**Honeydew melon wedge**

---

# Grilled Sirloin

*Total preparation time: 15 minutes*

**Four 7-ounce lean sirloin steaks, about ¾ inch thick, trimmed of fat**

1. Prepare outdoor grill or set oven to broil.
2. Grill or broil steaks, turning once, 4 to 5 minutes per side, depending on thickness and desired degree of doneness. (To test for doneness, cut a slit and note color: pink indicates medium, gray indicates well-done. Or, using meat thermometer, medium is an internal temperature of 160°F, well-done is 170°F.) Remove from grill or broiler and allow to rest 2 to 3 minutes before serving, for juices to set.

SERVES 4

# Garlicky Oven Fries

*Total preparation time: 30 minutes*

½ cup low-sodium chicken broth
1 teaspoon garlic powder
⅛ teaspoon ground black pepper
4 medium baking potatoes, scrubbed, dried, and cut lengthwise into
    ¼-inch-by-¼-inch-thick spears
Vegetable cooking spray

1.  Preheat oven to 400°F.
2.  In a large bowl, combine broth with garlic powder and black pepper. Add potato spears and toss to coat well.
3.  Spray a baking sheet with vegetable cooking spray. Arrange potatoes in a single layer, and bake 20 to 25 minutes, turning frequently, until crisp-tender.

SERVES 4

# Multicolored Salad

*Total preparation time: 12 minutes*

½ pound radicchio, washed and dried

½ pound arugula, washed and dried

1 head Bibb lettuce, outer leaves removed, washed, dried, and torn into
  bite-size pieces

1 head endive, washed, dried, separated into leaves

2 large carrots, peeled, tops and bottoms removed, cut into ¼-inch slices

½ cup fat-free raspberry vinaigrette dressing

Place greens in a large bowl and toss with carrots. Dress with vinaigrette.
Serve immediately.

SERVES 4

## NUTRITIONAL INFORMATION PER SERVING

|  | Calories | Protein | Carbohydrate | Fat | Fiber | Sodium | Cholesterol | Calcium |
|---|---|---|---|---|---|---|---|---|
| **Grilled Sirloin** | 258 | 42 g | 0 g | 9 g | 0 g | 115 mg | 121 mg | 14 mg |
| **Garlicky Oven Fries** | 139 | 3 g | 31 g | 0.5 g | 3 g | 23 mg | 0 mg | 15 mg |
| **Multicolored Salad** | 85 | 3 g | 18 g | 1 g | 3 g | 78 g | 0 mg | 127 mg |
| **Asparagus Spears** | 39 | 4 g | 8 g | 0.5 g | 3.5 g | 3 mg | 0 mg | 36 mg |
| **Parsley Carrot Coins** | 49 | 1 g | 12 g | 0 g | 3 g | 41 mg | 0 mg | 33 mg |
| **Honeydew melon wedge** **(⅛ melon)** | 56 | 1 g | 15 g | 0 g | 1 g | 16 mg | 0 mg | 10 mg |
| **Meal Total** | 626 | 54 g | 84 g | 11 g (16%) | 13.5 g | 276 mg | 121 mg | 235 mg |

Cajun Grilled Flank Steak
Grilled Zucchini
Small Baked Potato (page 226)
Corn on the Cob (page 180)
Fennel-Onion Salad (page 182)
Mango

# Cajun Grilled Flank Steak

*Total preparation time: 45 minutes*

2 teaspoons Cajun seasoning
2 cloves garlic, peeled and minced *or* 1 teaspoon prepared minced garlic
2 tablespoons low-sodium beef broth
1¾ pounds flank steak

1.   In a small bowl, combine Cajun seasoning, garlic, and beef broth. Rub steak with mixture, cover, and refrigerate 20 minutes.
2.   Meanwhile, prepare grill or set oven to broil. Grill or broil, turning once, 4 to 5 minutes per side, depending on thickness and desired degree of doneness. (To test for doneness, cut a slit and note color: pink indicates medium, gray indicates well-done. Or, using meat thermometer, medium is an internal temperature of 160°F, well-done is 170°F.)
3.   Remove from grill or broiler and allow to rest 2 to 3 minutes, for juices to set. Slice steak thinly across the grain, and baste with cooking juices.

SERVES 4

# Grilled Zucchini

*Total preparation time: 10 to 15 minutes*

**4 large zucchini, tops and bottoms removed, scrubbed, and cut lengthwise into ¼-inch slices**
**½ cup fat-free salad dressing**

1.  Prepare grill or set oven to broil.
2.  Brush zucchini with dressing. Lay slices directly on grill, or broil in a shallow pan, until crisp-tender, 5 to 10 minutes.

SERVES 4

NUTRITIONAL INFORMATION PER SERVING

|  | Calories | Protein | Carbohydrate | Fat | Fiber | Sodium | Cholesterol | Calcium |
|---|---|---|---|---|---|---|---|---|
| **Cajun Flank Steak** | 417 | 54 g | 1 g | 20 g | 0 g | 404 mg | 133 mg | 17 mg |
| **Grilled Zucchini** | 47 | 2 g | 11 g | 0 g | 2 g | 16 mg | 0 mg | 29 mg |
| **Baked Potato** | 104 | 2 g | 24 g | 0 g | 2.5 g | 49 mg | 0 mg | 17 mg |
| **Corn on the Cob** | 83 | 3 g | 19 g | 1 g | 2 g | 13 mg | 0 mg | 2 mg |
| **Fennel-Onion Salad** | 74 | 3 g | 17 g | 0.5 g | 4 g | 54 mg | 0 mg | 79 mg |
| **Mango (½ cup)** | 54 | 0.5 g | 14 g | 0 g | 1.5 g | 2 mg | 0 mg | 8 mg |
| **Meal Total** | 779 | 64.5 g | 86 g | 21.5 g (25%) | 12 g | 538 mg | 133 mg | 152 mg |

Greek-Style Burrito
Tomato-Cucumber Salad
Steamed Green Beans (page 224)
Diet gelatin

## Greek-Style Burrito

*Total preparation time: 30 to 40 minutes*

⅔ cup uncooked white rice
1¾ pounds extra-lean (91%) ground beef
4 small cloves garlic, peeled and minced
½ teaspoon dried mint
½ teaspoon dried oregano
½ teaspoon cumin
¼ teaspoon salt
¼ cup plain nonfat yogurt
Four 6-inch flour tortillas, warmed (see Note)
½ head iceberg lettuce, outer leaves removed, washed, dried, and shredded

1. Place rice and 1⅓ cups water in medium saucepan. Cover and bring to a boil. Reduce heat to low and simmer 14 minutes. Do not stir or lift cover. Remove from heat and let rice steam, covered, an additional 10 minutes.
2. Meanwhile, brown beef and garlic in a large nonstick skillet over medium-high heat. Drain on paper towels to remove all fat.
3. Return meat-garlic mixture to skillet and add mint, oregano, cumin, and salt. Cook over medium heat 1 minute, stirring constantly.
4. Remove from heat. Stir in yogurt and cooked rice, mixing well. Spoon onto center of warm tortilla, top with shredded lettuce, and roll up.

SERVES 4

Note: To warm tortillas in the microwave, place flat in microwave and heat on medium 45 to 50 seconds until hot; do not overheat. *Oven method*: Wrap tortillas in aluminum foil and warm in 250°F oven 10 minutes.

# Tomato–Cucumber Salad

*Total preparation time: 8 minutes*

4 medium tomatoes, washed and sliced
4 medium cucumbers, peeled and thinly sliced
½ cup fat-free salad dressing
4 large pieces of red- or green-leaf lettuce, washed and dried

1. Place tomatoes and cucumbers in a medium bowl and toss with salad dressing.
2. Place one piece of lettuce on each of four salad plates and top with equal portions of the tomato-cucumber mixture.

   SERVES 4

NUTRITIONAL INFORMATION PER SERVING

|  | Calories | Protein | Carbohydrate | Fat | Fiber | Sodium | Cholesterol | Calcium |
|---|---|---|---|---|---|---|---|---|
| **Greek-Style Burrito** | 632 | 49 g | 57 g | 22 g | 3 g | 394 mg | 73 mg | 78 mg |
| **Tomato-Cucumber Salad** | 93 | 4 g | 20 g | 0.5 g | 5 g | 22 mg | 0 mg | 74 mg |
| **Steamed Green Beans** | 35 | 2 g | 8 g | 0 g | 4 g | 7 mg | 0 mg | 42 mg |
| **Diet gelatin (1 cup)** | 20 | 4 g | 2 g | 0 g | 0 g | 0 mg | 0 mg | 0 mg |
| **Meal Total** | 780 | 59 g | 87 g | 22.5 g (26%) | 12 g | 423 mg | 73 mg | 194 mg |

Veal Chops with Papaya Salsa
White Rice
Parsley Carrot Coins (page 163)
Steamed Pea Pods
Steamed Green Beans
Melon chunks with sliced kiwi

# Veal Chops with Papaya Salsa

*Total preparation time: 20 minutes*

Nonstick cooking spray
Four ½-pound veal chops, with bone, ¾ inch thick (or four 6-ounce
    boneless chops)
1 large ripe papaya, peeled and chopped
One 6-ounce can crushed pineapple (water-packed or in juice)
1 teaspoon chopped fresh cilantro
1 teaspoon lime juice

1. Spray a large nonstick skillet with cooking spray. Sauté veal chops over medium-high heat 6 minutes on each side, or until cooked through, and internal temperature reads 160°F.
2. Meanwhile, combine papaya, pineapple, cilantro, and lime juice in a large bowl. Mix well.
3. Place cooked chops on serving platter and top with papaya salsa.

SERVES 4

# White Rice

*Total preparation time: 25 minutes*

**⅔ cup uncooked white rice**
**¼ teaspoon salt**

Place rice, salt, and 1⅓ cups water in medium saucepan. Cover and bring to a boil. Reduce heat to low and simmer 14 minutes. Do not stir or lift cover. Remove from heat and let rice steam, covered, an additional 10 minutes.

SERVES 4

# Steamed Pea Pods

*Total preparation time: 12 minutes*

**1 pound fresh pea pods, ends removed, stringed and washed**

1.  Fill a large saucepan with 2 inches water and set to boil.
2.  Place pea pods in steamer or colander and place in saucepan. Steam vegetables 5 minutes, or until crisp-tender.

SERVES 4

# Steamed Green Beans

*Total preparation time: 12 minutes*

**1 pound fresh green beans, ends removed and washed**

1.  Fill a large saucepan with 2 inches water and set to boil.
2.  Place beans in steamer or colander and place in saucepan. Steam 5 minutes, or until crisp-tender.

SERVES 4

NUTRITIONAL INFORMATION PER SERVING

|  | Calories | Protein | Carbohydrate | Fat | Fiber | Sodium | Cholesterol | Calcium |
|---|---|---|---|---|---|---|---|---|
| **Veal Chops** <br> **with Papaya Salsa** | 410 | 53 g | 13 g | 14 g | 2 g | 133 mg | 193 mg | 79 mg |
| **White Rice** | 105 | 2 g | 23 g | 0 g | 0.5 g | 0 mg | 0 mg | 3 mg |
| **Parsley Carrot Coins** | 49 | 1 g | 12 g | 0 g | 3 g | 41 mg | 0 mg | 33 mg |
| **Steamed Pea Pods** | 48 | 3 g | 9 g | 0 g | 3 g | 5 mg | 0 mg | 49 mg |
| **Steamed Green Beans** | 35 | 2 g | 8 g | 0 g | 4 g | 7 mg | 0 mg | 42 mg |
| **Melon chunks (1 cup)** <br> **with sliced kiwi ($^1\!/_2$)** | 79 | 2 g | 19 g | 0.69 g | 3 g | 16 mg | 0 mg | 28 mg |
| **Meal Total** | 717 | 63 g | 84 g | 15 g (19%) | 15.5 g | 202 mg | 193 mg | 234 mg |

---

**Mint-Glazed Lamb Chop**
**Baked Potato**
**Asparagus Spears**
**Red Beets**
**Tossed Salad (page 162)**
**Honeydew melon wedge**

---

# Mint-Glazed Lamb Chop

*Total preparation time: 25 minutes*

**4 teaspoons cornstarch**
**$^1\!/_4$ cup snipped fresh mint *or* 2 teaspoons dried**
**3 tablespoons light corn syrup**
**1 teaspoon grated lemon peel, yellow part only (with no white pith)**
**Four 7-ounce lamb chops, $^3\!/_4$ inch thick, trimmed of fat**

1.   Preheat oven to broil.
2.   In a small saucepan, stir $^1\!/_2$ cup water with the cornstarch. Add mint, corn syrup, and grated lemon peel. Simmer over medium heat, stirring contin-

ually, 3 to 5 minutes, until thick and bubbly. Cook an additional 2 minutes. Remove from heat and set aside.

3.  Place lamb chops on broiler pan 3 inches from heat, and cook 4 minutes. Brush with half the glaze. Turn, brush with remaining glaze, and broil 4 to 5 minutes for medium, or until the internal temperature is 160°F.

SERVES 4

# Baked Potato

*Total preparation time: 10 or 65 minutes, depending on method*

**2 large russet or Idaho baking potatoes, with skin, well-scrubbed**
**4 tablespoons salsa**

*Oven method:* Preheat oven to 400°F. Prick each scrubbed potato a few times with a fork. Place on a baking sheet and cook 50 to 60 minutes, or until soft when pricked by a fork. Cut in half and top each serving with 1 tablespoon salsa. *Microwave method:* Prick scrubbed potatoes with a fork twice. Place side by side on a paper towel in center of microwave oven. Cook on high 5 to 8 minutes, or until soft when pricked by a fork. Cut in half and top each serving with 1 tablespoon salsa.

SERVES 4

# Asparagus Spears

*Total preparation time: 10 minutes*

**1½ pounds asparagus, ends removed and rinsed**

1.  Fill a large saucepan with 2 inches water and set to boil.
2.  Steam asparagus spears in colander over boiling water until crisp-tender, 6 to 8 minutes.

SERVES 4

# Red Beets

*Total preparation time: 30 minutes*

**1½ pounds fresh red beets, with skins, washed**

1. Fill a large saucepan with 3 cups water (enough to cover the beets) and set to boil. Cook beets for 20 minutes or until tender when pierced by a fork. Drain and allow to cool.
2. When beets are cool enough to handle, peel and slice. Serve warm.

SERVES 4

NUTRITIONAL INFORMATION PER SERVING

|  | Calories | Protein | Carbohydrate | Fat | Fiber | Sodium | Cholesterol | Calcium |
|---|---|---|---|---|---|---|---|---|
| **Mint-Glazed Lamb Chop** | 393 | 47 g | 14 g | 15 g | 0 g | 151 mg | 149 mg | 35 mg |
| **Baked Potato** | 104 | 2 g | 24 g | 0 g | 2.5 g | 49 mg | 0 mg | 17 mg |
| **Asparagus Spears** | 39 | 4 g | 8 g | 0.5 g | 3.5 g | 3 mg | 0 mg | 36 mg |
| **Red Beets** | 75 | 3 g | 17 g | 0 g | 1 g | 122 mg | 0 mg | 27 mg |
| **Tossed Salad** | 88 | 5 g | 18 g | 1 g | 5 g | 35 mg | 0 mg | 73 mg |
| **Honeydew melon wedge (⅛ melon)** | 56 | 1 g | 15 g | 0 g | 1 g | 16 mg | 0 mg | 10 mg |
| **Meal Total** | 755 | 62 g | 96 g | 16.5 g (20%) | 13 g | 376 mg | 149 mg | 198 mg |

# Breakfasts

Most people find that Slim•Fast shakes and bars are best enjoyed for breakfast and lunch, with a sensible dinner rounding out the day. But for those days when it's easiest to take along a shake for lunch and dinner—or for those days when you just would rather have a full plate of breakfast in front of you—here are some perfect options:

---

**Blueberry Whole Wheat Pancakes**
**topped with powdered sugar, 1 tablespoon**
**Sliced fresh strawberries, 1/2 cup**
**Fat-free milk, 1/2 cup**
**Coffee, 1 cup, with artificial sweetener**

---

## Blueberry Whole Wheat Pancakes

*Total preparation time: 20 minutes*

3/4 cup all-purpose flour
3/4 cup whole wheat flour
2 teaspoons baking powder
4 teaspoons granulated sugar
2 egg whites
1 3/4 cups skim milk
1 tablespoon canola oil
1 cup blueberries, rinsed
Nonstick cooking spray

1. In a small bowl, combine all-purpose flour, whole-wheat flour, baking powder, and sugar. Mix well and set aside.

2.  In a large bowl, combine egg whites, milk, and oil. Add flour mixture and stir until just moistened and lumpy. Gently fold in blueberries.

3.  Spray a large nonstick skillet with cooking spray and set over medium heat. For each pancake, spoon about 3 tablespoons batter into the hot pan, making a small circle. Cook until pancakes are bubbly on top, 4 minutes. Flip and cook until browned on bottom, 2 to 3 additional minutes.

SERVES 4

NUTRITIONAL INFORMATION PER SERVING

|  | Calories | Protein | Carbohydrate | Fat | Fiber | Sodium | Cholesterol | Calcium |
|---|---|---|---|---|---|---|---|---|
| **Blueberry Whole Wheat Pancakes** | 275 | 11 g | 49.5 g | 4 g | 4 g | 330 mg | 2 mg | 281 mg |
| **Powdered sugar** | 24 | 0 g | 6 g | 0 g | 0 g | 0 mg | 0 mg | 0 mg |
| **Strawberries** | 25 | 0.5 g | 6 g | 0.5 g | 2 g | 1 mg | 0 mg | 12 mg |
| **Fat-free milk** | 40 | 4 g | 5.5 g | 0.2 g | 0 g | 58 mg | 2 mg | 139 mg |
| **Meal Total** | 364 | 15.5 g | 67.0 g | 4.7 g | 6 g | 389 mg | 4 mg | 432 mg |

Apple Oat Bran Muffin
Orange juice, ½ cup
Cantaloupe wedge, ⅛ melon
Low-fat cottage cheese with pineapple, ½ cup
Coffee, 1 cup, with artificial sweetener and 2 ounces fat-free milk

## Apple Oat Bran Muffins

*Total preparation time: 30 minutes*

1 medium tart apple (Granny Smith or McIntosh), peeled, cored, and thinly
   sliced
1 tablespoon lemon juice
1¼ cups white flour
1 cup oat bran
1 tablespoon baking powder
1½ teaspoons ground cinnamon
¼ teaspoon ground nutmeg
1 cup unsweetened prepared applesauce
½ cup skim milk
¼ cup firmly packed brown sugar
1 egg white
2 tablespoons shortening replacement (applesauce or other prepared
   replacement)
½ cup raisins

1.  Preheat oven to 425°F. Line ten 2½-inch muffin cups with cupcake papers.
2.  In a small bowl, toss apple slices with lemon juice and set aside. In a large
    bowl, combine flour, oat bran, baking powder, cinnamon, and nutmeg. In
    a separate bowl, mix applesauce, milk, sugar, egg white, shortening

replacement, raisins, and the apple slices with lemon juice. Combine the wet and dry ingredients, and mix well.

3.   Spoon the batter into muffin cups and bake at 425°F 15 to 20 minutes, or until a toothpick inserted in center of muffins comes out clean.

MAKES 10 MUFFINS

NUTRITIONAL INFORMATION PER SERVING

|  | Calories | Protein | Carbohydrate | Fat | Fiber | Sodium | Cholesterol | Calcium |
|---|---|---|---|---|---|---|---|---|
| **Apple Oat Bran Muffin** | 133 | 4 g | 32 g | 1 g | 3 g | 161 mg | 0 mg | 112 mg |
| **Orange juice** | 51 | 1 g | 12 g | 0 g | 0 g | 1 mg | 0 mg | 12 mg |
| **Cantaloupe wedge** | 24 | 1 g | 6 g | 0 g | 0.5 g | 6 mg | 0 mg | 8 mg |
| **Cottage cheese** | 110 | 11 g | 11 g | 1.5 g | 0 g | 291 mg | 10 mg | 40 mg |
| **Fat-free milk** | 20 | 2 g | 3 g | 0 g | 0 g | 29 mg | 1 mg | 70 mg |
| **Meal Total** | 338 | 19 g | 64 g | 2.5 g | 3.5 g | 488 mg | 11 mg | 242 mg |

Peach-Berry Crumble
Orange juice, ½ cup
Nonfat yogurt, artificially sweetened, 6 ounces
Coffee, 1 cup, with artificial sweetener and 2 ounces fat-free milk

## Peach–Berry Crumble

*Total preparation time: 1 hour*

1 tablespoon cornstarch
1 teaspoon ground cinnamon
½ teaspoon ground nutmeg
½ cup granulated sugar
2 pounds fresh peaches, washed, pitted, and thinly sliced
1 cup blueberries, rinsed
1 cup all-purpose baking mix (such as Bisquick)
¼ cup margarine
1 egg

1. Preheat oven to 375°F.
2. In a shallow, 1½- to 2-quart baking dish, mix cornstarch, cinnamon, nutmeg, and ¼ cup of the sugar. Gently stir in peaches and blueberries.
3. In a food processor or large bowl, combine remaining ¼ cup sugar, baking mix, and margarine. Whirl (or mix) until mixture has the coarse texture of cornmeal. Add egg and stir until just blended.
4. Sprinkle the batter mixture evenly over the fruit mixture. Bake in 375° oven until top is golden, about 45 minutes.

SERVES 8

NUTRITIONAL INFORMATION PER SERVING

|  | Calories | Protein | Carbohydrate | Fat | Fiber | Sodium | Cholesterol | Calcium |
|---|---|---|---|---|---|---|---|---|
| **Peach-Berry Crumble** | 231 | 4 g | 41 g | 7 g | 3 g | 245 mg | 27 mg | 39 mg |
| **Orange juice** | 51 | 1 g | 12 g | 0 g | 0 g | 1 mg | 0 mg | 12 mg |
| **Nonfat yogurt** | 70 | 7 g | 11 g | 0 g | 0 g | 80 mg | 2.5 mg | 200 mg |
| **Meal Total** | 352 | 12 g | 64 g | 7 g (16%) | 3 g | 336 mg | 29.5 mg | 251 mg |

Spicy Turkey Breakfast Sausage

Honeydew wedge, 1/8 melon

Whole wheat toast, 1 slice

Reduced–calorie fruit spread, 1 tablespoon

Coffee, 1 cup, with artificial sweetener and 2 ounces fat-free milk

# Spicy Turkey Breakfast Sausage

*Total preparation time: 15 minutes*

1/2 small onion, peeled, finely diced

1 pound ground, skinned turkey breast

1 teaspoon chopped fresh rosemary *or* 1/2 teaspoon dried

2 teaspoons chopped fresh sage *or* 1 teaspoon dried

1/2 teaspoon black pepper

1. Place onion in small bowl and cover with Saran Wrap. Microwave on high (100 percent power) 45 seconds. In a large bowl, combine turkey, rosemary, sage, and pepper. Add onions and mix well. Form into 8 patties, each 3 inches in diameter and 1/4 inch thick.

2. Place patties in large nonstick skillet and cook over high heat 1 minute; turn and cook 1 more minute. Reduce heat to low and cook, turning occasionally, until golden brown and cooked through, 3 more minutes.

SERVES 4

NUTRITIONAL INFORMATION PER SERVING

| | Calories | Protein | Carbohydrate | Fat | Fiber | Sodium | Cholesterol | Calcium |
|---|---|---|---|---|---|---|---|---|
| Spicy Turkey Breakfast Sausage | 176 | 20 g | 1.5 g | 9 g | 0.5 g | 107 mg | 90 mg | 23 mg |
| Honeydew wedge | 56 | 1 g | 15 g | 0 g | 1 g | 16 mg | 0 mg | 10 mg |
| Whole wheat toast | 69 | 3 g | 13 g | 1 g | 2 g | 148 mg | 0 mg | 20 mg |
| Reduced-calorie fruit spread | 20 | 0 g | 5 g | 0 g | 0 g | 20 mg | 0 mg | 0 mg |
| Meal Total | 321 | 24 g | 34.5 g | 10 g (19%) | 3.5 g | 291 mg | 90 mg | 53 mg |

**Easy Oven–Baked Hash Browns**
**Grapefruit half**
**Scrambled eggs (egg substitute),**
**½ cup (made with nonstick cooking spray)**
**Fat-free milk, 6 ounces**
**Coffee, 1 cup, with artificial sweetener**

# Easy Oven–Baked Hash Browns

*Total preparation time: 35 minutes*

1 teaspoon paprika
½ teaspoon black pepper
1 tablespoon canola oil
1½ pounds russet potatoes, unpeeled, scrubbed, and cut into ½-inch-thick
    wedges

1.   Preheat oven to 450°F.
2.   In a small bowl, combine paprika and pepper. Lightly brush 2 baking
    sheets with ½ tablespoon of the oil. Arrange potato wedges on the baking

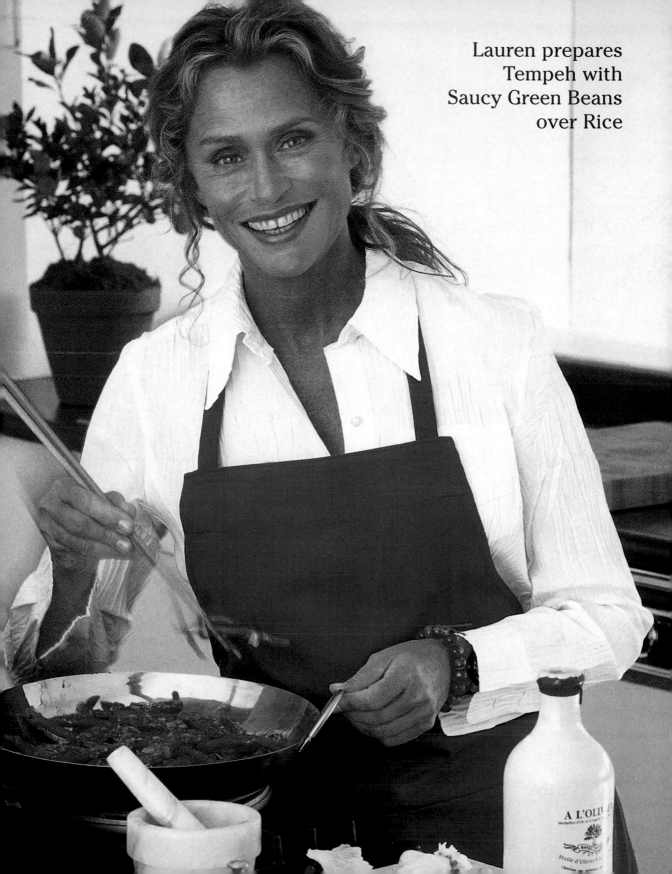

Lauren prepares
Tempeh with
Saucy Green Beans
over Rice

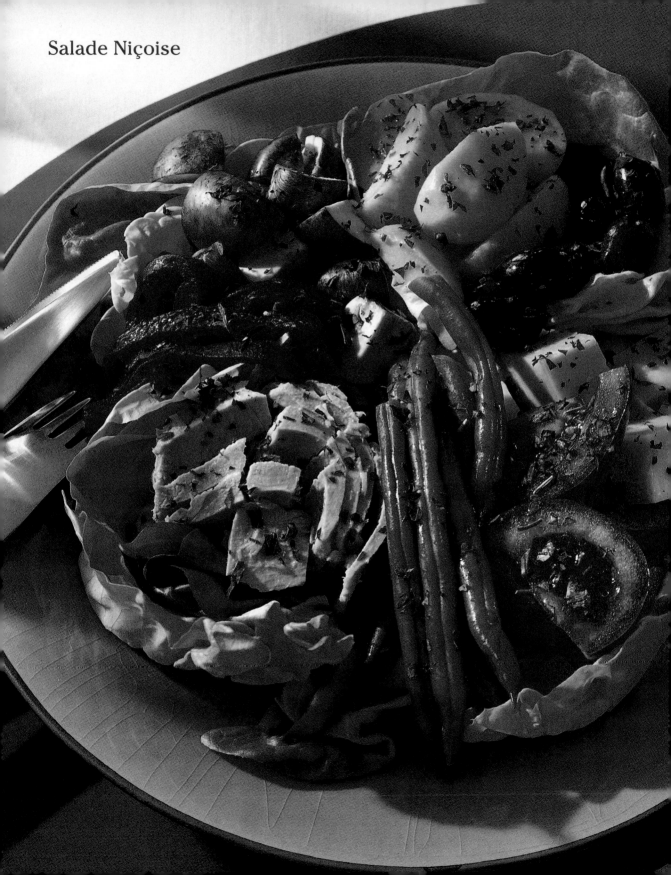

Salade Niçoise

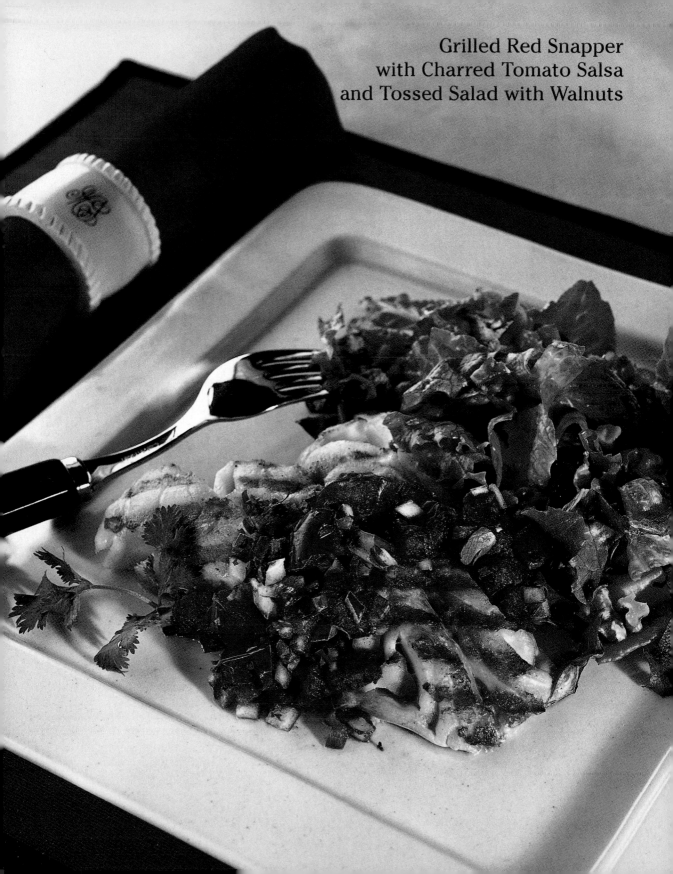

Grilled Red Snapper
with Charred Tomato Salsa
and Tossed Salad with Walnuts

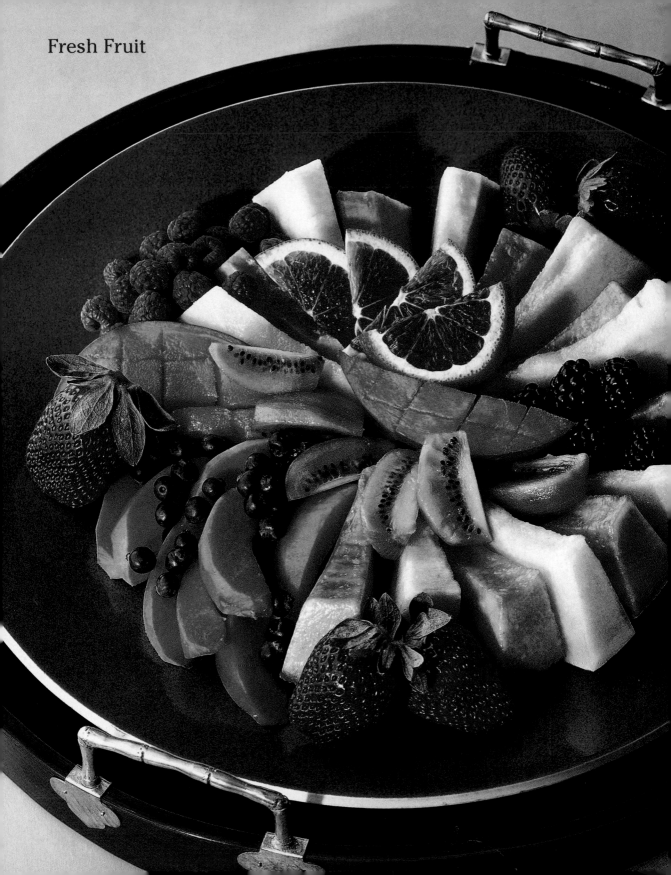

Fresh Fruit

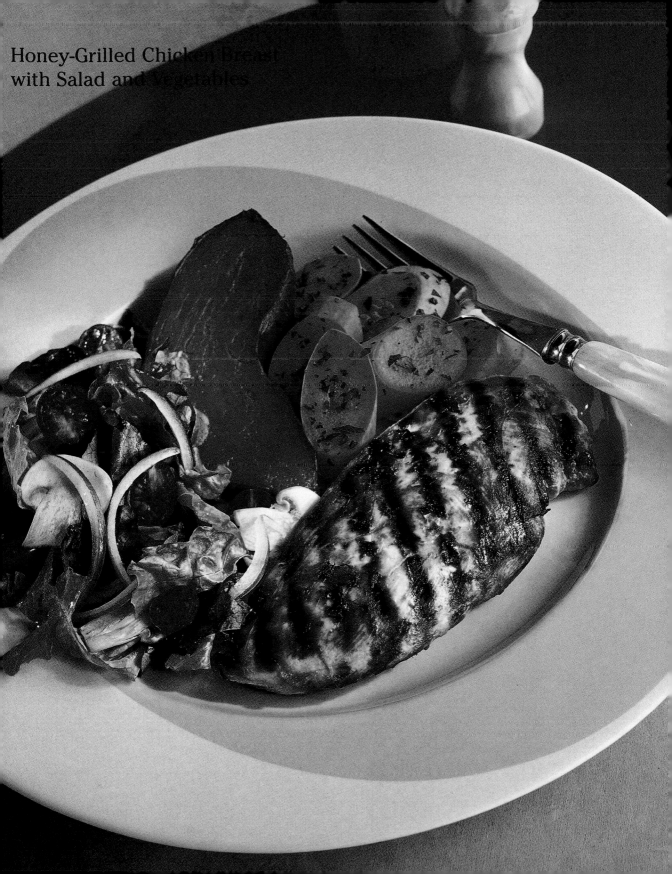

Honey-Grilled Chicken Breast
with Salad and Vegetables

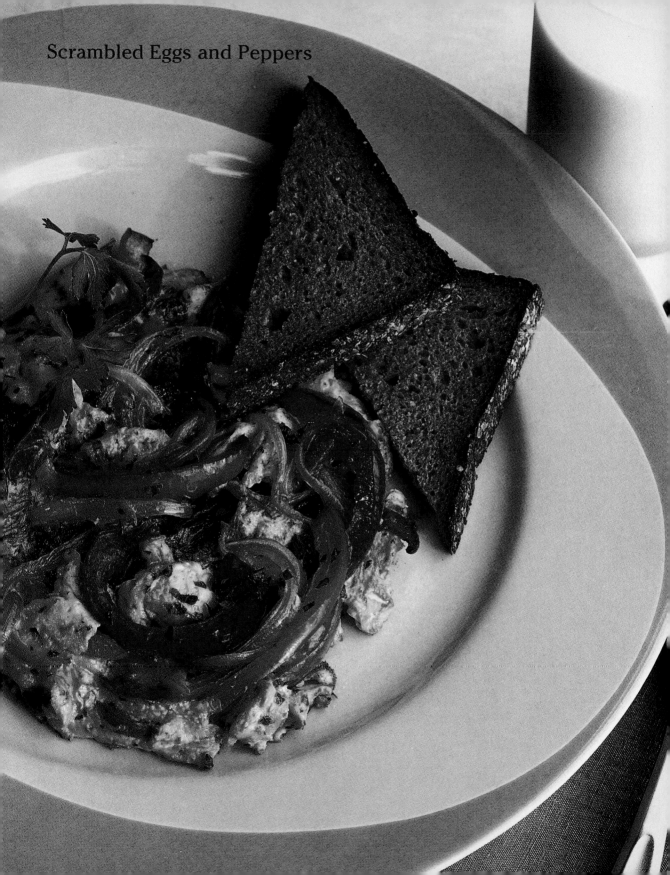

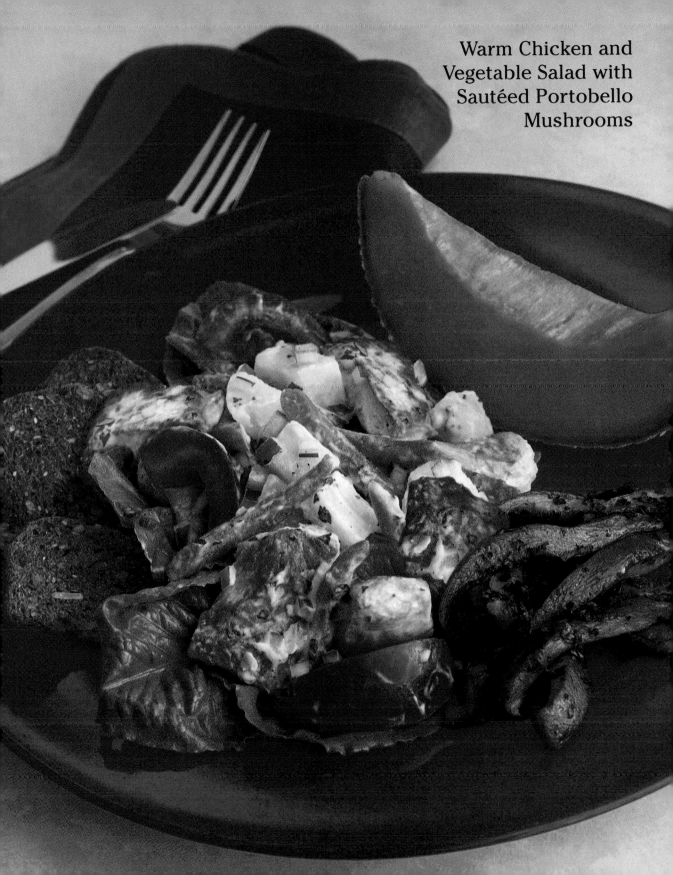

Warm Chicken and Vegetable Salad with Sautéed Portobello Mushrooms

# Diving is exhilarating . . .

Taking the plunge into that lagoon is like falling backward into
Botticelli's clamshell, arms outstretched—Venus laughing . . .

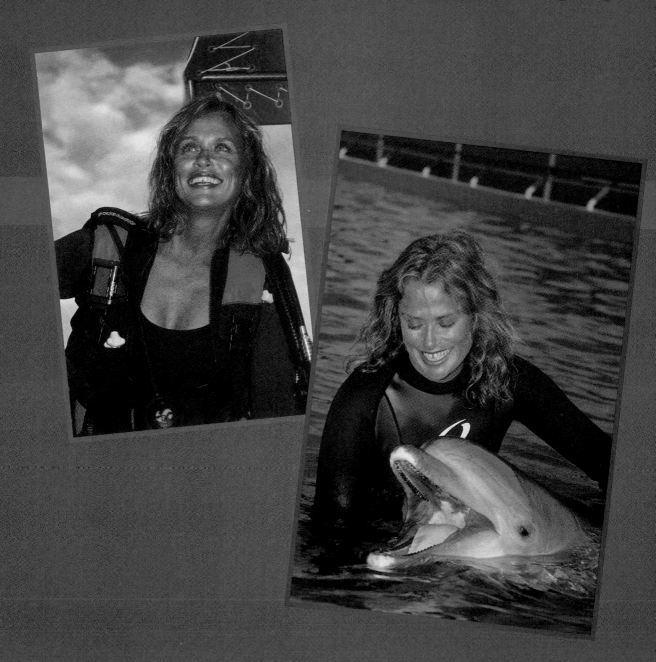

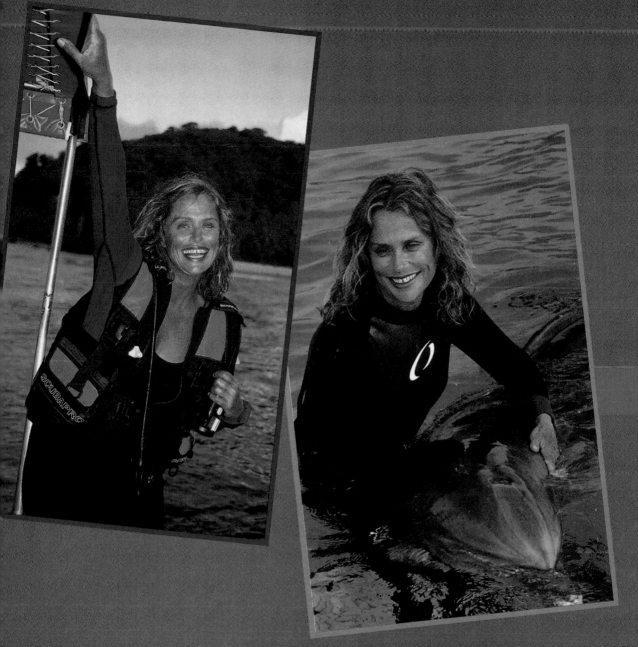

But it's also tough business. When you're scurrying around more than a hundred feet below the surface, you realize how important it is to be in shape.

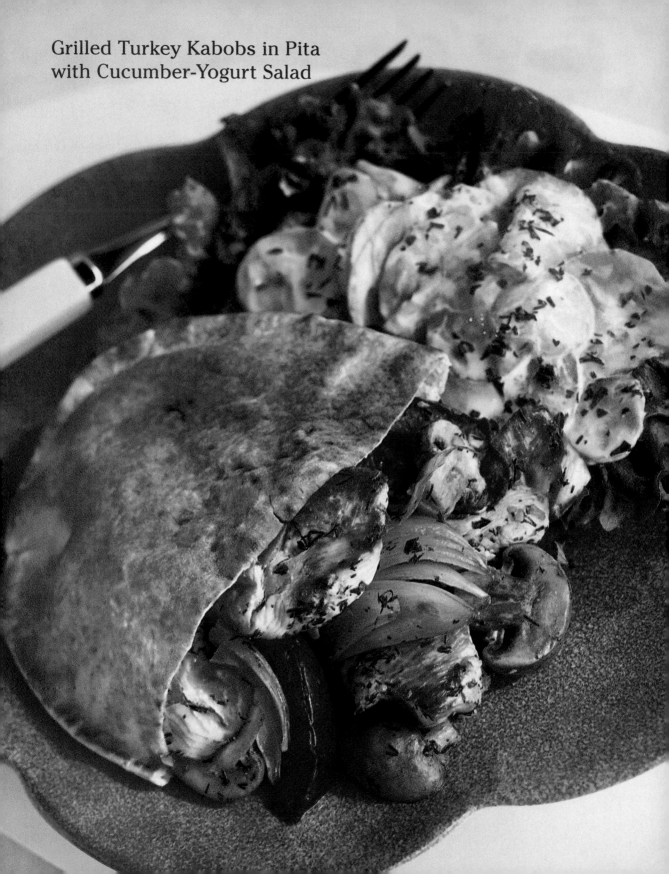

Grilled Turkey Kabobs in Pita
with Cucumber-Yogurt Salad

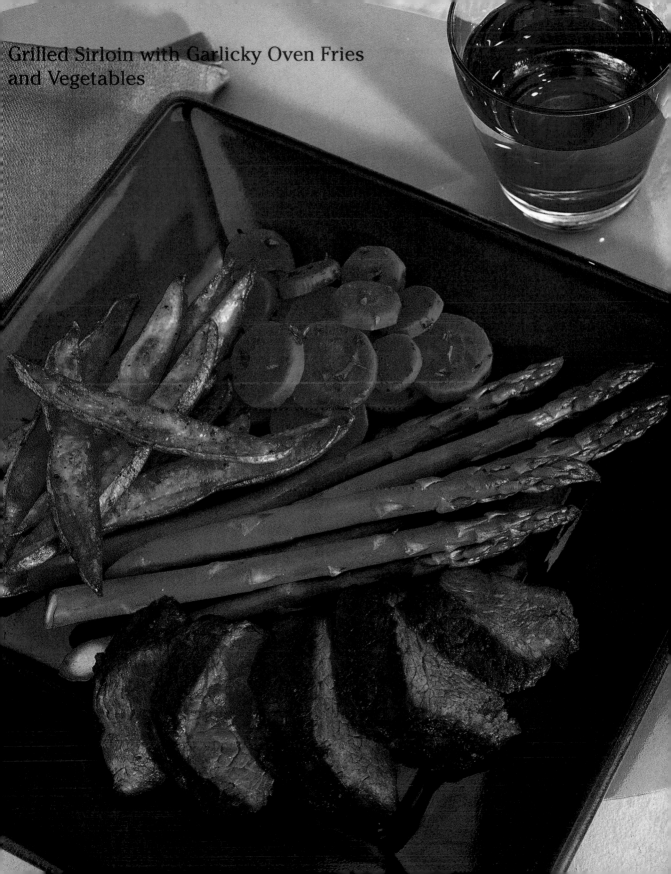

Grilled Sirloin with Garlicky Oven Fries
and Vegetables

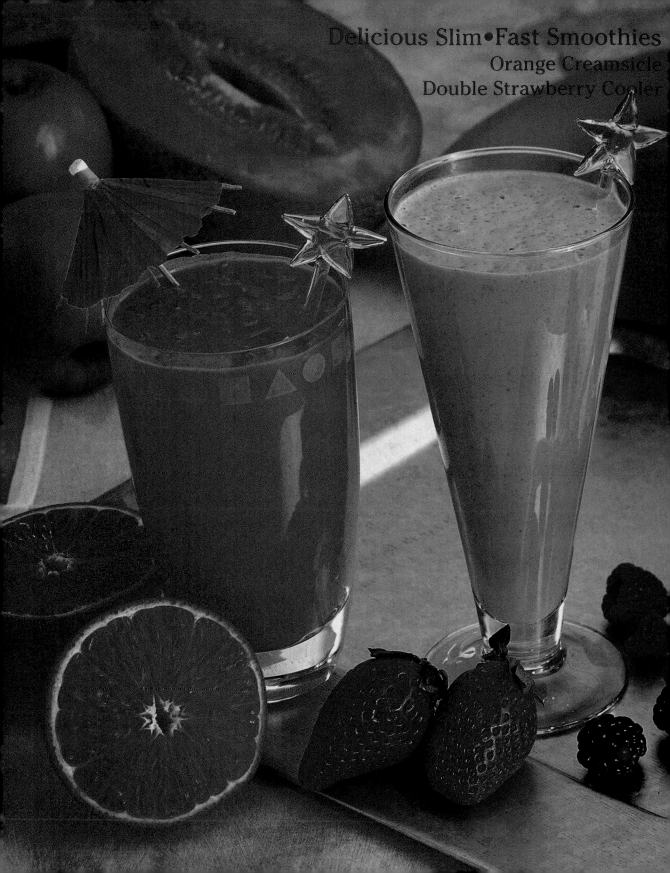

Delicious Slim•Fast Smoothies
Orange Creamsicle
Double Strawberry Cooler

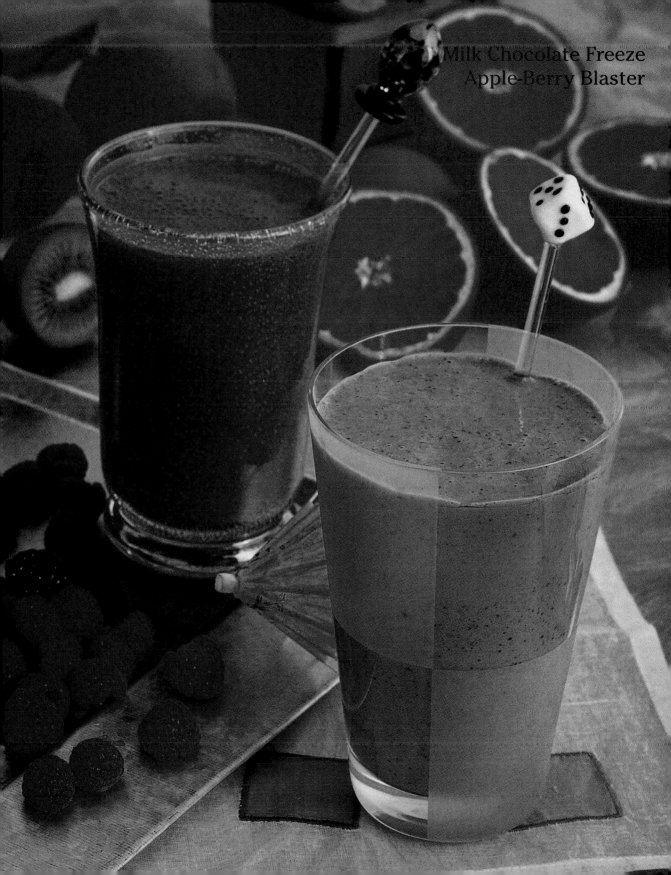

Milk Chocolate Freeze
Apple-Berry Blaster

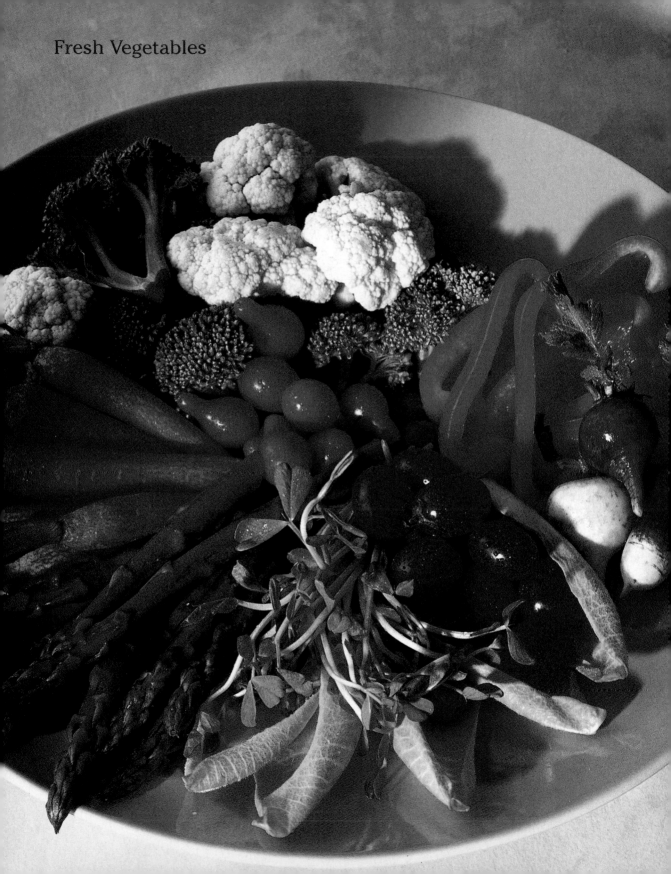

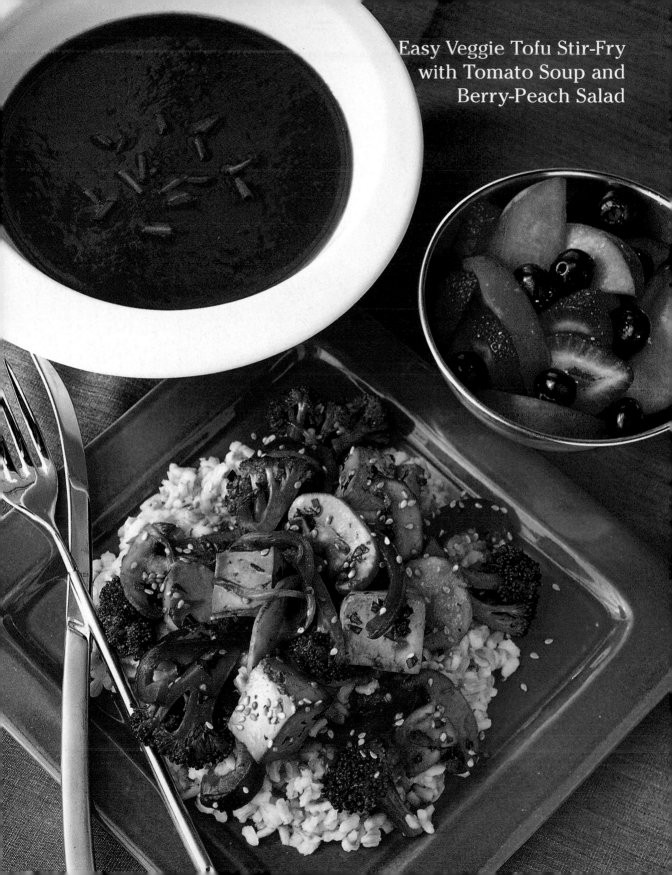

Easy Veggie Tofu Stir-Fry
with Tomato Soup and
Berry-Peach Salad

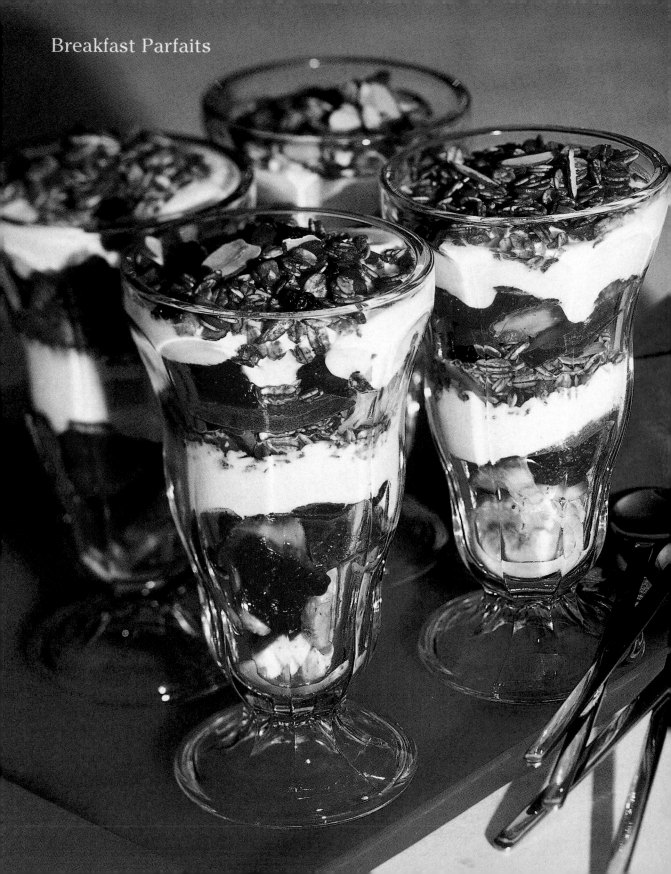

Breakfast Parfaits

sheets, brush with half the remaining oil, and sprinkle with half the paprika mixture.

3.  Bake at 450°F for 15 minutes. Turn, brush with the remaining oil, and sprinkle with remaining paprika mixture. Continue to bake until golden brown, 10 more minutes.

SERVES 4

NUTRITIONAL INFORMATION PER SERVING

|  | Calories | Protein | Carbohydrate | Fat | Fiber | Sodium | Cholesterol | Calcium |
|---|---|---|---|---|---|---|---|---|
| **Easy Oven-Baked Hash Browns** | 14 | 2.5 g | 27 g | 4 g | 2 g | 6 mg | 0 mg | 8 mg |
| **Grapefruit half** | 37 | 1 g | 9 g | 0 g | .5 g | 0 mg | 0 mg | 18 mg |
| **Egg substitute** | 106 | 15 g | 1 g | 4 g | 0 g | 222 mg | 1 mg | 67 mg |
| **Fat-free milk** | 59 | 6 g | 8 g | 0.5 g | 0 g | 88 mg | 3 mg | 209 mg |
| **Meal Total** | 216 | 24.5 g | 45 g | 8.5 g (20%) | 2.5 g | 316 mg | 4 mg | 302 mg |

**Scrambled Eggs and Peppers**
**Whole-grain toast, 1 slice**
**Fresh orange, 1 medium**
**Bran flakes, ½ cup**
**Fat-free milk, 6 ounces**
**Coffee, 1 cup, with artificial sweetener**

# Scrambled Eggs and Peppers

*Total preparation time: 20 minutes*

1 teaspoon olive oil
1 medium onion, peeled and thinly sliced
1 medium green pepper, washed, cored, seeded, and thinly sliced
1 medium red bell pepper, washed, cored, seeded, and thinly sliced
1 medium yellow bell pepper, washed, cored, seeded, and thinly sliced
1½ cups egg substitute
2 tablespoons skim milk
½ cup chopped fresh parsley

1. Heat the olive oil in a large nonstick skillet over medium-high heat. Add onion and cook, stirring frequently, until wilted, 5 minutes.
2. Add sliced peppers and cook 1 minute. Cover and continue to cook until peppers are soft, 2 more minutes.
3. Meanwhile, in large bowl, beat together egg substitute, milk, and parsley. Pour over pepper mixture, reduce heat to medium, and cover. Cook until egg mixture is lightly firm, 2 minutes.

SERVES 4

## NUTRITIONAL INFORMATION PER SERVING

|  | Calories | Protein | Carbohydrate | Fat | Fiber | Sodium | Cholesterol | Calcium |
|---|---|---|---|---|---|---|---|---|
| **Scrambled Eggs and Peppers** | 119 | 12 g | 7 g | 4 g | 2 g | 175 mg | 1 mg | 75 mg |
| **Whole-grain toast** | 69 | 3 g | 13 g | 1 g | 2 g | 148 mg | 0 mg | 20 mg |
| **Orange** | 62 | 1 g | 15 g | 0 g | 3 g | 0 mg | 0 mg | 52 mg |
| **Bran flakes** | 63 | 2 g | 15 g | 0.5 g | 3 g | 151 mg | 0 mg | 9 mg |
| **Fat-free milk** | 59 | 6 g | 8 g | 0.5 g | 0 g | 88 mg | 3 mg | 209 mg |
| **Meal Total** | 372 | 24 g | 58 g | 6 g (15%) | 10 g | 562 mg | 4 mg | 365 mg |

# Specialty Shakes and Smoothies

One of the great things about Slim•Fast shakes is that you can dress them up so many different ways. This selection of recipes represents only a few of the delicious health drinks that can be made quickly and easily with Ultra Slim•Fast shakes and powders. Don't feel limited to this list—it's just a start! Get creative; invent your own sensational shakes and smoothies based on your favorite ingredients and flavor combinations—Mocha Mint, Chocolate Almond Fudge, Cocoa-Banana, or Banana Berry. Experiment and share your great-tasting recipes with a friend. The healthy possibilities are endless!

The following recipes can be made in less than five minutes using nutrient-packed Ultra Slim•Fast powders. Try making creamy milk-based shakes and smoothies with the Chocolate Royale, Strawberry Supreme, or French Vanilla. Try the Fruit Juice mixer for icier, juice-based drinks.

## Cappuccino Smoothie

**1 heaping scoop Chocolate Royale Ultra Slim•Fast powder**
**1 cup fat-free milk, chilled**
**1 teaspoon instant coffee**
**6 ice cubes**

Blend all ingredients together in a blender for 40 seconds. Pour into a tall glass and enjoy.

NOTE: This smoothie can also be made by substituting 1 heaping scoop Vanilla Ultra Slim•Fast and 1 tablespoon chocolate syrup for the Chocolate Royale Ultra Slim•Fast.

## Chocolate Mint Shake

**1 heaping scoop Chocolate Royale Ultra Slim•Fast powder**
**1 cup fat-free milk, chilled**
**¼ teaspoon peppermint extract**
**4 ice cubes**

Blend all ingredients together in a blender for 40 seconds. Pour into a tall glass and enjoy.

## Quick Fudge Pops

1 heaping scoop Chocolate Royale Ultra Slim•Fast powder
1 cup fat-free milk, chilled
1 teaspoon cocoa powder
1 packet sugar substitute
4 ice cubes

1. Blend all ingredients together in a blender for 40 seconds. Pour into three 4-ounce paper cups or plastic Popsicle molds. Place in freezer.
2. When pops are half-frozen (about 15 minutes) insert Popsicle sticks. Let freeze completely.
3. To unfreeze, peel away the paper cup or run warm water on the outside of the Popsicle mold. Enjoy!

MAKES THREE 4-OUNCE POPS

## Milk Chocolate Freeze

1 heaping scoop Chocolate Royale Ultra Slim•Fast powder
2 teaspoons cocoa powder
¾ cup fat-free milk, chilled
2 packets sugar substitute
¼ teaspoon vanilla extract
10 ice cubes

1. Combine all ingredients in a blender and blend for 40 seconds. Transfer to a metal mixing bowl and place in freezer for about 2 hours.
2. Remove frozen mixture from freezer and let sit 10 minutes. Transfer contents back to the blender and blend until smooth. Serve immediately.

## Double Strawberry Cooler

1 heaping scoop Strawberry Supreme Ultra Slim·Fast powder
1 cup fat-free milk, chilled
½ cup fresh or frozen strawberries
6 ice cubes

Blend all ingredients together in a blender for 40 seconds. Pour into a tall glass and enjoy.

## Strawberry Banana Sipper

1 heaping scoop Strawberry Supreme Ultra Slim·Fast powder
1 cup fat-free milk, chilled
½ banana, peeled and cut into slices
4 ice cubes

Blend all ingredients together in a blender for 40 seconds. Pour into a tall glass and enjoy.

## Orange Creamsicle

1 heaping scoop Vanilla Ultra Slim·Fast powder
½ cup orange juice, chilled
½ cup fat-free milk, chilled
½ cup plain nonfat yogurt
4 ice cubes

Blend all ingredients together in a blender for 40 seconds. Pour into a tall glass and enjoy.

## Vanilla Tapioca Pudding

1 tablespoon instant tapioca
1 cup fat-free milk
1 heaping scoop French Vanilla Ultra Slim•Fast powder
½ teaspoon vanilla extract
A pinch of ground nutmeg

1. Combine tapioca and milk in saucepan. Let sit 5 minutes. Cook mixture over medium heat, stirring frequently until mixture reaches a full boil.
2. Remove from heat, transfer to a blender, add the Slim•Fast and vanilla extract. Blend 30 seconds on medium speed.
3. Let cool at room temperature for 20 minutes for warm tapioca, or refrigerate until cool for chilled tapioca. Sprinkle with nutmeg before serving.

## Apple Berry Blaster

1 heaping scoop Ultra Slim•Fast Fruit Juice powder
1 cup orange juice or apple juice, chilled
¼ cup frozen blueberries
¼ cup frozen strawberries
6 ice cubes

Blend all ingredients together in a blender for 40 seconds. Pour into a tall glass and enjoy. For a thicker, icier smoothie, add 2 more ice cubes.

## Tropical Breeze

1 heaping scoop Ultra Slim•Fast Fruit Juice powder
1 cup orange or orange/pineapple juice, chilled
3 slices canned pineapple
4 ice cubes

Blend all ingredients together in a blender for 40 seconds. Pour into a tall glass and enjoy.

## Raspberry Refresher

1 heaping scoop Ultra Slim·Fast Fruit Juice powder
1 cup apple juice
½ cup frozen unsweetened raspberries
1 packet sugar substitute
4 ice cubes

Blend all ingredients together in a blender for 40 seconds. Pour into a tall glass and enjoy.

## Sunrise Shake

1 can Ultra Slim·Fast French Vanilla Ready-to-Drink Shake, chilled
¼ cup fresh or frozen peaches, cut into chunks
¼ cup fresh or frozen strawberries
6 ice cubes

Blend all ingredients together in a blender for 40 seconds. Pour into a tall glass and enjoy.

## Chocolate–Dipped Strawberry Shake

1 can Ultra Slim·Fast Rich Chocolate Royale Ready-to-Drink Shake, chilled
½ cup frozen strawberries
6 ice cubes

Blend all ingredients together in a blender for 40 seconds. Pour into a tall glass and enjoy.

## Cherry Vanilla Shake

1 can Ultra Slim·Fast French Vanilla Ready-to-Drink Shake, chilled
½ cup canned or frozen black cherries (be sure to select the no-sugar
  variety)
1 teaspoon vanilla extract
6 ice cubes

Blend all ingredients together in a blender for 40 seconds. Pour into a tall glass and enjoy.

## Breakfast Parfaits

*Total preparation time: 10 minutes*

1 pint strawberries, hulled, rinsed, and sliced
2 bananas, peeled and sliced
4 peaches or nectarines, washed, pitted, and sliced
2 packets sugar substitute (optional)
4 cups nonfat vanilla yogurt, artificially sweetened
1 cup fat-free granola

1.  In a large bowl, combine berries, bananas, and peaches. For tart fruit, sprinkle with sugar substitute if desired.
2.  Spoon ⅓ cup of the fruit mixture into each of 4 parfait or other tall glasses; pat down lightly to create an even layer. Top each with ⅓ cup yogurt and sprinkle with 1 tablespoon granola. Repeat with another layer each of fruit, yogurt, and granola.
3.  Top the glasses with the remaining fruit, add a dollop of the remainning yogurt, and sprinkle with granola. Serve immediately.

SERVES 4

# 7

# YOUR EXERCISE AND
# RELAXATION MAKEOVER

Now that you've read all about the eating plan, you may be tempted to focus just on changing your eating habits and skipping the rest of the Body•Mind•Life Makeover. After all, if you've dieted before, that's probably all you did—put different kinds or smaller amounts of food into your mouth. But you know how successful that was, right?

So now it's time to do things differently. It's time to make changes that will actually enrich your life—enabling you to have a healthier, more adventurous, and more enjoyable life. And that's what the makeover is all about: putting both your body and your mind on the right track. Of course, it's possible to lose weight simply by eating better for a limited period of time; but if you want to keep the weight off for good—and look and feel as good as you should—you've got to change your mind-set and lifestyle as well.

After giving yourself the makeover, you'll no longer feel compelled to park in the closest parking space, or take a people mover in the airport to save yourself the walk. You'll be less tempted to use food to ease your boredom or help you cope with a stressful day. You'll find that you obsess less about food as you turn to other ways to relax and get enjoyment out of life.

This chapter will help you create your own exercise plan and develop your own relaxation plan. These are the very components that are usually missing from diet plans, but they're essential for upping the odds of success. They work hand in hand to combat food cravings and improve your overall well-being. For instance, combining exercise and relaxation can ease the PMS munchies and mood swings, and help you through a stressful period at work—two things that can sabotage even the best-laid weight-loss plans. In terms of your body chemistry, both exercise and relaxation lower your body's level of stress hormones and boost your level of chemicals such as endorphins and serotonin, which can make you feel happy and calm. Both are also great for your health and may help lower your risk of heart disease and other illnesses.

Countless Slim•Fast users have found that exercise is a key component in weight loss. They've also found that exercise and weight loss build on each other: Losing weight improves your ability to exercise and enables you to do activities you may never have thought you could manage. Andy Fisher of Gainesville, Florida, says:

> I first realized I needed to lose weight when I struggled to get into my wet suit before a planned scuba dive. I wrestled with it and wrestled with it, but I couldn't zip it up. It was an embarrassing moment. I was in shock.
>
> Going through the Slim•Fast Plan, I felt like I was going through a whole cleansing cycle. I was actually cleaning out my body and learning to eat properly and take care of myself. Since going on the plan, I lost over 43 pounds and have been able to keep it off for six months. There are things I can do now that I never thought possible—like going on a thirty-mile bike ride or hiking to the top of a mountain. Now I follow a regular exercise routine and have a shake at least once a day. It's a true joy to wake up in the morning and know that you're going to have a lot of energy and going to be able to tackle anything that comes your way.

After you've read through the exercises on the following pages, it's your turn to use them as the building blocks of your own exercise program. The Makeover Diary at the back of the book will give you a place to keep track of every new exercise you try, and help you learn more about what kind of workout will work best for you.

# Creating Your Personal Exercise Plan

Exercise, of course, is key to successful weight loss; combined with a balanced diet, it can help you take off weight and create a more toned and efficient body. And yet many people have spent years shying away from physical activity. Beginning an exercise program can be daunting—especially if you don't know enough about what to do.

This plan is designed to teach you the basics. You will learn three different types of exercises—aerobic activity, resistance training, and stretching—all of which your body needs. You'll become stronger, feel more energy, and develop a firmer, fitter body. Exercise can be just as easy as changing your eating habits. What's more, once you see how good it makes you feel, you'll find you can't live without it.

If you're already following a workout program, feel free to continue the exercises that are working for you—but you can also use this as an opportunity to try something new. Buy yourself a new workout video, or take the spinning class that you always wanted to try at the gym. You may learn something from the advice in the following pages: Maybe you're not stretching as much as you should, or you're neglecting to strengthen your muscles through resistance training.

This plan will show you that exercise doesn't need to make you grunt and groan to be beneficial. It sweeps aside the "no-pain-no-gain" philosophy in favor of exercise in moderation—an approach supported by recommendations from prestigious groups such as the American College of Sports Medicine and the Centers for Disease Control and Prevention, which emphasize that moderate amounts of activity can provide health benefits and weight loss to people who previously were sedentary.

On this plan you'll have a simple goal: Get one hour of exercise per day. As we've discussed, this isn't as difficult as it sounds—especially if you accumulate activity throughout the day. Walk fifteen minutes each way to take your child to school every morning, and you'll only need thirty minutes on the exercise bike in the evening.

If you've never exercised before and you are severely overweight, it'll probably take you several weeks before you can handle sixty minutes of activity each day. That's okay. Work your way up slowly. Start with a fifteen-minute walk on the first day, and gradually increase the time as your stamina increases. What's important to realize is that any amount of exercise is beneficial. More exercise is better than some, and some is better than none.

Don't think of exercise as a formal regimen you're forcing yourself to follow until you lose the weight and you can give it up. Like the Slim•Fast eating plan, the exercise plan is a life change that you'll want to stay with because it makes you feel good. You just need to allow yourself a few weeks to get into the exercise groove. If you have to skip a workout one day, don't beat yourself up about it. Just find ways to add little bursts of activity into your days, like taking the stairs at work instead of the elevator. Even forgoing those electronic gadgets—TV remote controls, automatic garage door openers, electric can openers—can help you burn up to 200 to 300 extra calories a day! The important thing is to stay committed.

## Making Exercise—and Love—a Part of Your Life

For me, exercise is always very tough to start, especially with my schedule constantly changing. When I first started trying to work a serious exercise regimen into my life, I had to start all over again time after time; I'd get going with a new gym regimen, then work would take me off somewhere else, and I'd get thrown off my rhythm. The big problem was, every time I stopped I felt I was reverting to ground zero; it was as if everything I'd done so far was for nothing, and I'd feel that old familiar depression creeping in, slow but steady.

Now I realize that the problem wasn't with me—it was with the inflexible, unrealistic demands I was trying to impose on my life. That's why the Slim•Fast program puts so much emphasis on creating a personal program that works for you. Whether it's going to the gym, doing aerobics at home, or simply taking a good hard walk through your neighborhood every day, what's most important isn't what kind of exercise you do—it's that you get it done.

Now I'm as faithful to my goals as I can be, but I don't chastise myself if I miss a day. And what always draws me back to my personal exercise plan is remembering how good I feel about my *self*—about my self-image—when I'm exercising regularly. And when I come back to it, after a couple of days it's like magic—I breathe better, think better, sleep better, and have infinitely more energy. Above all, I *like* myself better, and maybe for good reason—because, for all of the above reasons, I'm a kinder and better person when I'm taking care of myself.

And don't forget about sex! I don't know if you're the same way, but when I'm not getting enough exercise, the last thing I'm interested in is the idea of sharing my unclothed, unfit body with my lover. Yikes! But after a few days of exercise, all those negative feelings are Hoovered away. Suddenly I'm full of optimism, peace of mind, and positive energy. And *voilà!* When you feel that way, your whole life is enhanced. And suddenly you have so much energy you feel like sharing it with others; next thing you know, you're interested, you're caring—and you're *sexy*. You twinkle for them. And you start sharing your joy . . . the sexiest feeling of all.

## Step 1: Get Your Calorie Burn

Steady or aerobic exercise—like walking, biking, running, and swimming—makes your body burn calories quickly, helping you shed excess pounds. It also strengthens your heart and helps build muscle. You'll probably also notice that you feel energized and invigorated after a workout—a boost researchers attribute to increases in the brain's level of endorphins.

It's time to choose an aerobic activity that you'll be comfortable doing on a regular basis, four or five days a week. If you haven't exercised before, you should choose a simple activity like walking or riding on a stationary bike. Once you've improved your fitness level, you can try a kick-boxing class or take tennis lessons. Unless you're in good physical shape, be aware that your first few weeks of exercise will be tough. You'll probably be huffing and puffing after just a few minutes of exertion, and you may not be having much fun as you try to get your body to do things it isn't used to.

As you build your endurance, though, you'll be amazed as your body's capabilities grow before your eyes. Where you could once barely manage a ten-minute walk, you'll find within weeks that a thirty-minute walk becomes a piece of cake.

Here are a few suggestions you can use as a guide for choosing an aerobic activity. After a brief description of each activity, you'll find recommended stretches you should do before and after your workouts. Instructions and illustrations for these stretches are found in the stretching section in Step 2. You'll also find the calculated calorie burn that you'll get from doing an hour of each activity. The calculation is based on a 150-pound person; if you weigh more you'll burn more calories, if you weigh less you'll burn less. Remember: Your goal is to get about an hour of activity each day, to burn an estimated 250 to 300 calories.

## AEROBICS

Aerobics is a combination of dance and calisthenics, and includes such variations as step aerobics, slide aerobics, and movement classes influenced by everything from jazz to hip-hop to funk. Classes like Tae-Bo and kick-boxing include moves from boxing, martial arts, and military boot-camp exercises.

**Benefits to your body:** Aerobics helps tone muscles throughout your entire body while burning calories at the same time, so you get more bang for your buck. It's also great for weight loss because it keeps you moving constantly, which burns more calories.

**It's easy:** You can learn techniques from the class or video instructor, so you don't need to be physically fit to begin. What's more, you can progress to a more advanced class or video, so you don't get bored if the workouts get too easy.

**Format:** Most aerobics classes and videos include a short warm-up and stretching period, a thirty-minute workout, stretching and cool-down, and a short muscle-toning session.

**What you'll need:** Sneakers with ankle support designed specifically for aerobics, or cross-trainers. Most good sneakers cost around $45 to $80. Wear exercise clothes made from a synthetic material (not cotton), which will wick sweat away from your skin. A sports bra is essential for women.

**Warm-up and stretches:** Most aerobics classes and videos include a warm-up and stretches at the beginning of the workout. If they don't, march in place for about five to ten minutes before stretching. Be sure to stretch the following muscle groups after your warm-up to reduce your risk of injury and after your cool-down to reduce soreness and increase flexibility:

Quadriceps: large muscles in front of thighs
Hamstrings: large muscles in back of thighs
Gluteus: buttock muscles
Calves
Triceps: muscles in back of upper arms
Biceps: muscles in front of the arms

**Cool-down:** If your instructor fails to do one, walk around for five to ten minutes to allow your heart rate to descend gradually.

**Calorie burn:** 340 calories per hour, moderate intensity. (Calorie calculations are based on 150-pound person. If you weigh more, you'll burn more calories; if you weigh less, you'll burn less.)

## WALKING

Walking is one of the safest and healthiest exercises you can do. A recent study from Harvard University found that walking briskly for three hours a week can cut the risk of heart disease in women by as much as 40 percent—equivalent to the benefits of regular aerobics, jogging, or other vigorous physical activity. Walking is also the cheapest, easiest form of exercise. All you have to do is open your door and get moving!

**Benefits to your body:** Walking strengthens the hips, thighs, butt, and legs. The faster your pace, the more calories you burn. The longer you walk, the more you build up your endurance. Besides reducing your risk of heart disease, walking may lower high blood pressure. And walking two or more miles a day can help older people live longer, according to a recent study. Walking also helps prevent osteoporosis, since it's a weight-bearing activity. Of course, it's also a great way to lose weight!

**It's convenient**: You can do it just about anywhere, at home on the treadmill or outdoors to get you to and from work. Whether you're alone or with friends, you can adjust your pace for almost any fitness level. To get a good workout, though, walk as briskly as you can. You should be breathing hard and sweating without feeling discomfort. Since it's easy on the joints, you can walk even if injury keeps you from more strenuous activity.

**Warm-up and stretches**: Go at about half speed for the first five minutes of your walk to allow your muscles to warm up. Be sure to stretch the following muscle groups after your warm-up to reduce your risk of injury and after your cool-down to reduce soreness and increase flexibility:

Quadriceps
Gluteus
Hamstrings
Calves

**Cool-down**: Slow your pace at the end of the walk to allow your heart rate to descend gradually.

**Calorie burn**: 272 calories per hour, brisk pace of 3.5 mph (based on 150-pound person).

## BIKING

Getting out and riding is one of the fastest ways to get physically fit. Even if you haven't biked in years, the cliché holds true—you never forget how.

**Benefits to your body**: Biking works your leg muscles, butt, and calves. And a recent study found that cycling for just thirty minutes six times a month may reduce the risk of premature death by more than half. Cycling is also gentle on the body and ideal for people who have joint or back problems.

**It's a mode of transportation**: You can bike to your errands or to work, so it's easy to fit in workouts. You can also plan biking vacations and use your bike to get to beautiful weekend retreats. To stay in shape in between biking jaunts, take a spinning class at the gym or ride a stationary bike at home.

**What you need**: A road bike, mountain bike, or hybrid bike. (You can buy one or rent one from a bike shop.) Bikes range from $150 up to $500. A road bike has thinner tires and a lighter frame, so it's easier to achieve speed. A mountain bike is heavier, lets you sit upright, and is less vulnerable to flat tires. Hybrid bikes let you sit upright and have sturdier wheels, but like road bikes, they're lighter. They're a good compromise for beginners. You also need a helmet to protect yourself from serious head injuries. Get one that's certified by the Consumer Products Safety Commission (CPSC). Wear comfortable clothes and sneakers.

**Warm-up and stretches**: Pedal at a comfortable pace for five to ten minutes until you break a light sweat. This will warm up your muscles. Be sure to stretch the following muscle groups after your warm-up to reduce your risk of injury and after your cool-down to reduce soreness and increase flexibility:

Calves
Gluteus
Hamstrings
Quadriceps
Upper and lower back

**Cool-down**: During the last few minutes of your ride, slow your pace to half-speed to let your heart rate descend gradually.

**Calorie burn**: 408 calories per hour, moderate intensity (based on 150-pound person).

## SWIMMING

Swimming is one of the few fitness activities that gives you a great workout without jarring your body. It's great for people of all fitness levels—especially beginners.

**Benefits to your body**: Along with strengthening your heart, it works your legs, arms, butt, and abdominal muscles. It's great for building stamina and muscle tone without overtaxing your joints.

**What you need**: A snug-fitting suit designed for athletic swimming, goggles to keep the chlorine out of your eyes, a swimming cap if your hair is ear-length or longer.

**Warm-up and stretches**: Get moving for five or ten minutes before you begin your workout. March in place, walk to the pool, or start out with slow, easy strokes. Be sure to stretch the following muscle groups after your warm-up to reduce your risk of injury and after your cool-down to reduce soreness and increase flexibility:

Quadriceps
Gluteus
Hamstrings
Calves
Triceps
Shoulders

**Cool-down**: When you're done, have a leisurely swim for a few minutes before getting out of the pool to give your muscles a chance to cool down.

**Calorie burn**: 544 calories per hour (based on 150-pound person).

## TENNIS

Tennis makes even a hard workout feel like a good time. Having a partner to compete with keeps you challenged, while your legs get a workout from a constant back-and-forth movement.

**Benefits to your body**: Tennis makes your joints more flexible, particularly in the hips and the shoulder used to serve. It also develops and tones your muscles, especially the quadriceps, hamstrings, calves, arms, shoulders, and upper back. As a bonus, you'll experience an improvement in hand-eye coordination, balance, and agility—and, of course, you'll get a cardiovascular workout.

**It's a social event**: Tennis is a great way to socialize. You can play with up to three other people at a time or sign up for round-robin tournaments. And you never have to forgo a tennis game because of the weather. Just take advantage of the abundance of indoor courts.

**What you need:** If you've never played tennis before, you should go to a certified teaching professional to learn the proper techniques for hitting the ball, so that you avoid injury. They can recommend the right racket for your playing style and skill level. Aerobic activities, strength training, and stretching will get you in the necessary condition for tennis.

**Warm-up and stretches:** You should warm up your muscles for five to ten minutes before playing to lower your risk of injury. Gently lob the ball back and forth a few times. Be sure to stretch the following muscle groups after your warm-up to reduce your risk of injury and after your cool-down to reduce soreness and increase flexibility:

Calves
Forearms
Gluteus
Hamstrings
Obliques
Quadriceps
Shoulders
Triceps
Upper and lower back

**Cool-down:** If you've played a light game, walk around the court to collect stray balls. If you've played intensely enough to get you sweating and breathing heavily, walk around until your heart rate returns to normal.

**Calorie burn:** 340 calories per hour (based on 150-pound person).

## SPINNING

Spinning, also called studio or indoor cycling, is offered as a group class in most gyms and is extremely challenging. With its loud music, dim lights, instructors shouting out orders, and the sound of many bikes working together, spinning has taken the fitness world by storm.

**Benefits to your body:** Spinning is an excellent way to lose weight because it burns a huge amount of calories. It tones your quadriceps, hamstrings, calves, hips, and abdominals. It also improves your cardiovascular fitness and endurance. During your first few weeks, though, you should take a spinning class for beginners; it's easy to overexert yourself trying to keep up with a pack of advanced spinners.

**It's low-impact and easier on the joints**: Compared to other high-intensity exercises like running and aerobics, spinning is low-impact and less likely to causes muscle injuries or joint problems. You may also find the team aspect appealing and fun. You should, however, be in moderately good physical shape. Any aerobic exercise like biking on your own time or walking can help you get in shape for a class.

**What you need**: Wear workout clothes made from a synthetic material to wick sweat away from your skin. Get a comfortable pair of bike shorts with padding in the seat area, which provides some needed cushioning. Have a towel on hand to mop up sweat from your face and hands.

**Warm-up and stretches**: Most instructors start with a warm-up, but if they don't, try a five-minute warm-up on a stationary bike before class yourself or take a brisk walk or jog. Be sure to stretch the following muscle groups after your warm-up to reduce your risk of injury and after your cool-down to reduce soreness and increase flexibility:

Quadriceps
Gluteus
Hamstrings
Calves

**Cool-down**: Allow your heart rate to descend gradually by walking around the studio or continuing to ride the stationary bike at a slow to moderately slow pace.

**Calorie burn**: 476 calories per hour (based on a 150-pound person).

## HIKING

Hiking is a great workout for all fitness levels if you enjoy the outdoors. Beginners can go on flat walks, while the experienced can head up a steep mountain. Almost every state park has trails that range from easy to challenging, at little or no cost to you.

**Benefits to your body:** As long as you keep up a steady pace, you can burn off a lot of calories and fat through hiking. Hiking will build your endurance and will help build muscle strength, particularly in the quadriceps, hamstrings, gluteus muscles, and calves. It will also strengthen your bones. Carrying a backpack will help you burn even more.

**It allows time for reflection:** Taking in the awe-inspiring beauty of nature will invigorate you and allow your mind to escape the stresses of daily life. Hiking also enables you to challenge your mind by plotting your own course and keeping yourself from getting lost. Hiking is a great group activity, though you may also enjoy it alone. If you're a solo hiker, be sure to tell someone where you're going and when you intend to get back in case you get lost or injured.

**What you need:** You'll need to invest in a pair of proper hiking boots. Ankle support is important—as is cushioning in the arch and heel, since trails can be rocky and uneven. Try on boots with the same socks you're planning to wear when you hike. Break in your new hiking boots at least a week before your trip. You also need a water bottle and an emergency kit in case you get lost (with extra food like a nutrition bar, water, a flashlight, a compass, a first-aid kit, and matches or a lighter).

**Warm-up and stretches:** Be sure to stretch the following muscle groups after your warm-up to reduce your risk of injury and after your cool-down to reduce soreness and increase flexibility:

Quadriceps
Gluteus
Hamstrings
Calves

**Cool-down:** Before you end your hike, slow down to a stroll for four or five minutes to allow your heart rate to descend gradually.

**Calorie burn:** 408 calories per hour (based on 150-pound person).

# Step 2: Stretch It to the Max

When you think about exercise, you probably don't think about stretching. Many exercisers neglect to stretch before and after workouts, writing it off as a waste of time. The truth is, although stretching itself doesn't directly contribute to weight loss, it has a host of other benefits. Stretching can enhance your performance during workouts by increasing your range of motion and improving your coordination; it can also help you avoid injuries that can sideline you for weeks.

Stretching for five to ten minutes before and after workouts can help avoid some of the ravages of aging—from decreased flexibility and poor balance to stiff joints. Regular stretching will relieve muscle tension, improve circulation, and enhance muscle tone. What's more, it makes you feel great!

A complete stretching routine appears below. It's best to warm up for three to five minutes before stretching to avoid pulling a muscle. Do any continuous movement that gets your heart rate elevated, like walking up and down the stairs a few times or jogging in place. *When you stretch, focus on the muscle being stretched and hold each stretch for ten to fifteen seconds. Repeat each stretch three to five times.* Try not to bounce, since this can force the joints past their natural range of motion, causing sprains of the ligaments or tendons. Stretch to a point where you feel a mild tension.

## Chest

Sit or stand with your hands clasped behind your back. With your hands intertwined, raise your hands upward a few inches until you feel mild tension between your shoulder blades and in your upper chest.

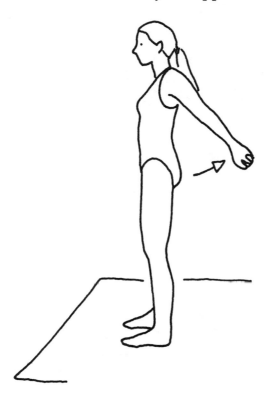

## Upper Back

Stand with your arms extended in front of you at shoulder height. Hold your hands together, fingers intertwined, with palms facing out. Round your shoulders and reach away from your chest. Keep your knees slightly bent throughout the stretch. You should feel the stretch across your entire upper back.

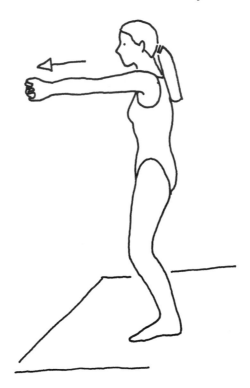

## Calves (opposite)

Stand with your hands and feet against a wall and take a large step back with one leg. Keep your legs aligned with your hips. With your front leg bent and your back leg straight, press the heel of your back leg into the floor. Press your hands into the wall for support, feeling the stretch in the back of your calf. Repeat on the other leg.

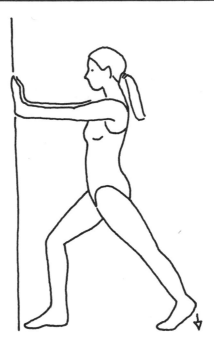

## Hamstrings (below)

Sit with your legs straight in front of you, with your feet relaxed (don't flex or point them). Bend one leg so that the bottom of your foot touches the inner thigh of the straight leg. Keeping your back straight and your chest out, bring your forehead toward the shin of the straight leg. Reach for your foot with both hands. Repeat on the other leg. You should feel this stretch in the back of your thigh. *Variation:* If you can't reach your foot, place a towel around your foot and hold on to the ends of the towel with both hands.

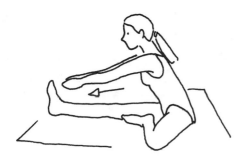 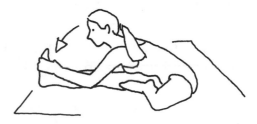

## Triceps

Sit or stand and extend both arms overhead. Bend one arm behind your head and push down on the elbow with the opposite hand. Repeat on the opposite arm. You should feel the stretch on the back of your upper arm.

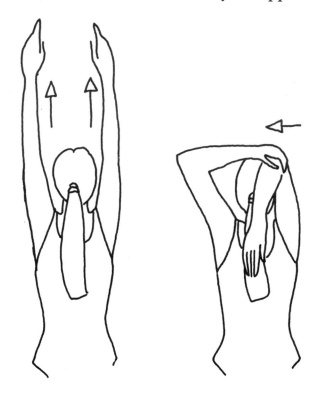

## Shoulders (opposite)

Place your right arm across your chest, keeping your arm straight and your shoulders down. Bring your left arm up from underneath, and place your left hand just above the right elbow. Pull your right arm gently toward your body. Repeat on the other side. You should feel the stretch across the top of your shoulder and upper arm.

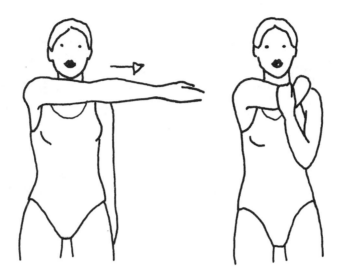

## Quadriceps (below)

Standing on your right leg, grab the ankle of your left leg with your left hand and pull your heel up behind you toward your buttock. Keep your knees close together and your back straight (not arched). Repeat on the other side. If you have sore knees, loop a towel around your ankle and keep your knee bent at a 90-degree angle. You should feel this stretch in the front of the thigh.

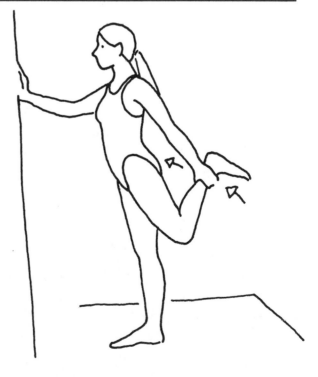

## Neck

Slowly drop your ear toward your right shoulder. When you reach a comfortable tension, gently lower your left shoulder. You should feel the stretch on the left side of your neck. Repeat the stretch on the other side. Now drop your chin toward your chest and hold. Keep your shoulders back. You should feel this stretch down the back of your neck and in your upper back.

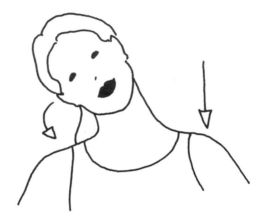

## Lower Back

Lie on your back with your knees bent and your feet flat on the floor. Keeping your knees bent, reach behind both legs under your thighs and bring your thighs into your chest, lifting your feet off the floor. Your lower back should remain on the floor. Your legs should feel relaxed through the entire move. You should feel this stretch in your lower back and buttocks.

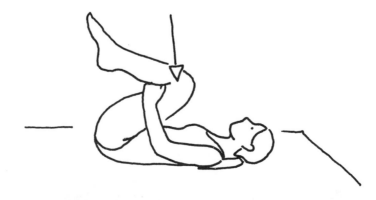

## Gluteus (Buttocks)

Lie on your back with both knees bent and your feet flat on the floor. Take your right foot in your left hand (wrapping your hand under your foot so that your fingertips are on its outside edge) and hold your leg (with your knee bent) in the air about one to three feet above your chest. Exhale and slowly pull your foot over to the side and up toward your head. You should feel the stretch in your buttocks. Repeat on the other side. If you have sore knees, wrap a towel around your ankle and use the ends of the towel to pull your leg up.

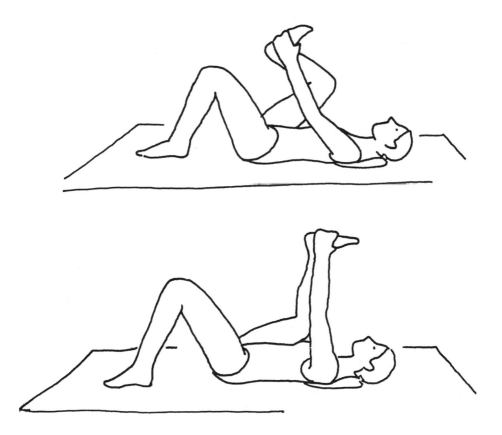

# Convenient Calorie Burners

Having trouble fitting a full hour of exercise into your daily routine? Here's a chart that highlights some simple and convenient exercises and activities that may be easier to fit into a busy day. Next to each activity is the calculated calorie burn (remember, you want to burn about 300 calories per day).

| Activity | Calories Burned (for 150-pound person) |
|---|---|
| Brisk walk around the block for 15 minutes | 68 |
| Sit-ups and push-ups for 10 minutes | 91 |
| Walking upstairs for 10 minutes | 91 |
| Dancing for 20 minutes | 93 |
| Cleaning your house for 30 minutes (vacuuming, mopping, dusting, cleaning bathrooms) | 119 |
| Light outdoor play with kids for 15 minutes | 68 |
| Lawn mowing for 40 minutes | 250 |
| Gardening for 20 minutes | 113 |
| Light snow shoveling for 30 minutes | 204 |
| Running in place for 10 minutes | 91 |
| Jumping rope slowly for 15 minutes | 136 |
| Shooting hoops for 20 minutes | 102 |

# Step 3: Pump Yourself Up

You've probably heard about the benefits of building muscle through strength or resistance training (the terms are synonymous). Resistance training makes you stronger and can make day-to-day tasks like hauling groceries much easier. It'll also make aerobic workouts much easier, as your muscles propel your body from place to place.

What you may not know is that strength training actually helps you burn more calories throughout the day, because muscle requires more calories to maintain than fat. Boosting your metabolism this way will help you lose weight and maintain the loss. In the long term, strength training can help prevent bone loss and protect against osteoporosis; it can also offset the increases in weight that usually occur with age as your metabolism starts to decline. Researchers from the University of Vermont in Burlington have found that lagging metabolism is due primarily to a loss of muscle mass from inactivity rather than to an inevitable metabolic meltdown.

You may have avoided strength training in the past out of fear of developing bulging muscles. But there isn't a very big risk of developing large muscles if you're doing the right amount of weight-lifting. What you should see is greater muscle definition and a sculpted look as your body gains tone. Unfortunately, though, you can't spot-reduce your stomach through abdominal crunches or your butt and thighs through squats. Aerobic activity will help burn off fat in all the areas of your body, while resistance training will give you a chiseled look.

If you don't have access to a gym's wide range of exercise machines, you'll need to get some basic equipment to get a full strength training workout. If you're just getting started, you can purchase a set of exercise (resistance) bands for about $20 in a sports equipment store. For weights, you can start by holding heavy soup cans or filled liter-size soda bottles. Once these weights get too light, you should purchase a set of dumbbells. A good starter set of dumbbells includes pairs of 2, 3, 5, 8, 10, 12, 15, and 20 pounds. You can buy a standard set of dumbbells for as little as $50 to $100, and you can even check the local classifieds for good deals.

The following exercises work all your major muscle groups. Aim to do this workout two to three times a week—though not on consecutive days, since muscles need a day to recover in between workouts.

One note: You may find that your rate of weight loss slows down as you begin to resistance-train. If you've been following your eating plan carefully, you're probably building muscle and lowering your percentage of body fat—which is, of course, a good thing. For reassurance, you can monitor your efforts by getting your body fat percentage tested—most health clubs offer these tests—but you should also be able to tell simply by monitoring your waistline and how well your clothes fit.

## Lunge

Works gluteus muscles, quadriceps, and hamstrings.

Stand with your feet together and your hands at your sides. Take an exaggerated step backward with your right leg.

Bend your right knee slowly, lowering your body close to the floor. Keep your right knee directly over your right foot and your back straight. Most of

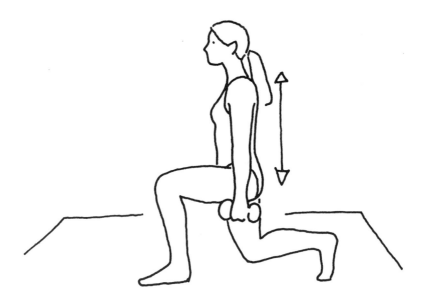

your weight will be over your right foot. You should feel the strain in your hips and thighs, not your knees, ankles, or back.

Hold position for one second and slowly return to starting position. Perform eight to twelve repetitions. Then do a set on your left leg.

**Variation:** Once you can do twelve repetitions with good form, you can make the exercise harder by holding a dumbbell in each hand.

**Weight room equivalent:** Leg press

## Knee Extension

Works your quadriceps.

Sit on a chair with your knees bent. Attach an exercise band to your right ankle and the rear leg of the chair. The band should be taut but not stretched.

Slowly lift your right foot, straightening your leg until it's parallel to the floor. Hold for one second.

Lower your foot back to the starting position. Do eight to twelve repetitions, then switch legs and repeat on the left leg.

**Variation**: Use ankle weights instead of exercise bands.

**Weight room equivalent**: Leg extension

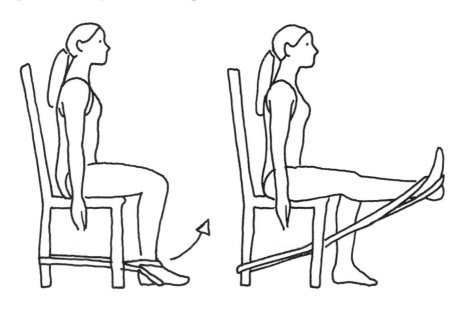

## Leg Curl

Strengthens your hamstrings.

Stand near a wall or a table. Attach one end of a resistance band to your right ankle and step on the other end with your left foot. To maintain your balance, place your feet no more than shoulder-width apart.

Keeping your knee still, bend your right leg and pull your foot as close to your buttocks as you can. Use the wall or table for support if necessary. Hold for one second, then slowly lower your foot to the ground.

Perform eight to twelve repetitions. Switch feet and do a set with your left leg.

**Variation:** Use ankle weights instead of exercise bands.

**Weight room equivalent:** Seated or prone leg curl

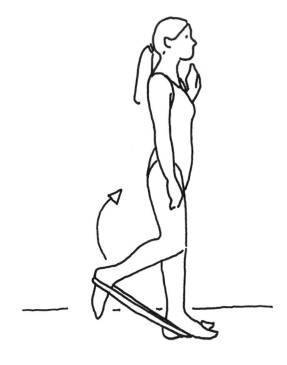

## Toe Raise

Works your calves.

Rest your hands on the back of a chair and position your feet straight in front of you about shoulder-width apart. Your toes should be facing forward or slightly outward.

Slowly raise your heels so that you're standing on the balls of your feet. Hold for one second. Slowly lower your heels to the ground. Do eight to twelve repetitions.

**Weight room equivalent:** Seated calf

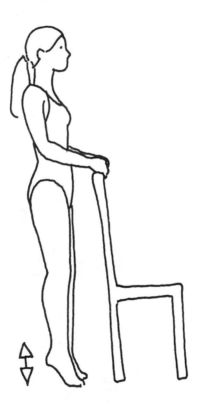

## Push-up

Works your chest muscles, as well as shoulder and triceps.

Lie face down on the floor with your hands flat on the floor, almost underneath your shoulders but a little wider apart.

Push your body off the floor, using your toes as a pivot point. Keep your back straight and your head in line with your body. (Beginners can do modified push-ups: Use your knees as the pivot point. Keep your toes on the floor or bend your knees at a 90-degree angle and cross your ankles.)

When your elbows are fully straightened, hold for one second. Slowly lower yourself to within one inch of the floor. You should feel the effort in your chest, shoulders, and triceps, not your neck. Without letting your chest touch the floor, do another push-up. Do eight to twelve repetitions.

**Weight room equivalent:** Bench press

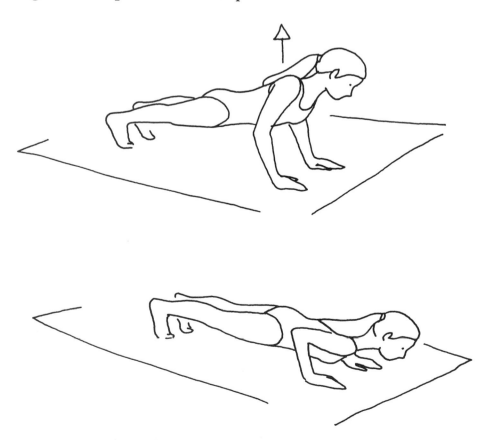

## Seated Row

Targets the upper back muscles.

Loop a resistance band around your feet. Sit on the floor with your legs straight in front of you. Grasp the ends of the band in your hands. It should have only slight tension.

Slowly pull your hands to your sides, pinching your shoulders together. Keep a relaxed but firm grip on the band. Your back should remain upright and your legs straight. You should feel the effort in your back, shoulders, and biceps.

Hold for one second. Slowly return your hands to the starting position. Perform eight to twelve repetitions.

**Weight room equivalent:** Seated or compound row

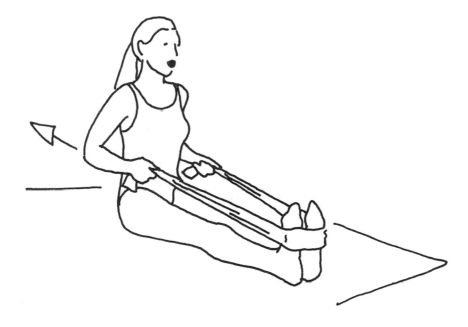

## Lateral Raise

Works the deltoid and rotator cuff muscles in the shoulders.

Standing with your arms at your sides and your feet shoulder-width apart, hold a dumbbell in each hand.

Keeping your arms straight and your palms facing in, lift your hands to the side to shoulder height. Keep your elbows slightly bent. You should feel the effort in your shoulders, not your neck or jaw.

Hold for one second, then slowly lower your arms back to your sides. Perform eight to twelve repetitions.

**Variation**: You can also do this exercise with an exercise band looped around each foot.

**Weight room equivalent**: Lateral raise machine

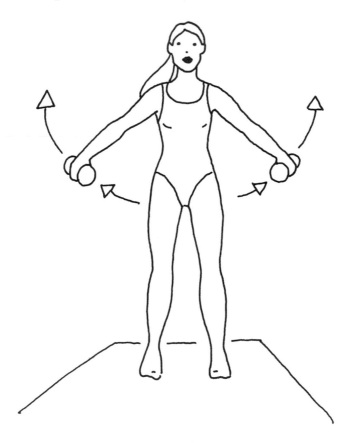

## Back Extension

Targets your lower back muscles.

Lie face down on the floor with your hands at your sides, next to your hips. Slowly raise your shoulders and chest off the floor about five inches by contracting your back muscles. Keep your lower body relaxed and your head in line with your upper body.

Hold for one second, then slowly lower your upper body to within one inch of the floor.

Perform eight to twelve repetitions.

**Weight room equivalent:** Lower back machine

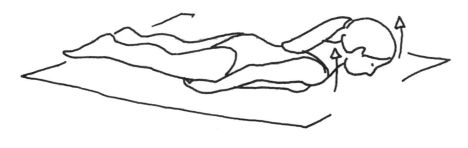

## Crunch

Works all your abdominal muscles.

Lie on the floor on your back with your knees bent at a 90-degree angle. Your feet should be flat on the floor. Cross your arms across your chest.

Slowly contract your abdominal muscles and raise your shoulder blades

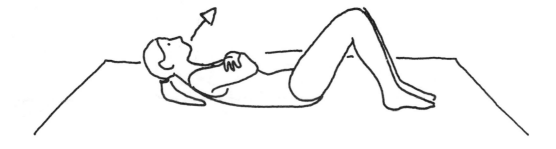

off the floor. Keep your head in line with your body—your chin off your chest, your neck relaxed. (Hint: Keep your eyes focused on your knees.)

Briefly hold this position, then slowly lower yourself back down to the floor. Do as many repetitions as you can while maintaining good form.

**Weight room equivalent:** Abdominal machine

## Arm Curl

Targets your biceps.

Stand upright with your arms at your sides, your feet about shoulder-width apart, and your knees slightly bent.

Grasp one end of the exercise band with your right hand, palm facing forward, and place your right foot on the other end. There should be a slight tension in the band.

Slowly bend your arm and bring your hand to your shoulder, keeping your elbow still and your back straight.

Hold for one second, and then slowly return to the starting position. Do eight to twelve repetitions, then repeat on your left side.

**Variation**: You can also do this exercise using a dumbbell instead of the exercise band.

**Weight room equivalent**: Arm curl, biceps curl, preacher curl

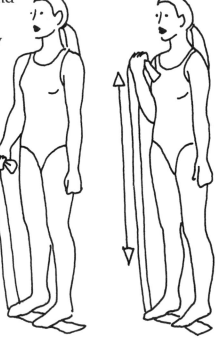

## Rear Extension

Works your triceps.

Stand to the right of a weight bench or behind a chair. Bend forward at the waist and place your left hand on the chair or bench. If you're using a bench, you can place your left knee on the bench for support.

Hold the dumbbell in your right hand, with your right elbow bent to a 90-degree angle and your upper arm next to your torso, parallel to the floor. Keep your palm facing in and the weight close to your side.

Straighten your arm in back of you to lift the weight, keeping your elbow and upper arm still. Don't twist your back or lock your elbow.

When your arm is straight behind you and parallel to the floor, pause for one second. Return to the starting position. Perform eight to twelve repetitions, then switch arms and repeat on the opposite side.

**Variation**: You can perform this exercise with a resistance band by stepping on one end with your foot and holding the other end in your hand.

**Weight room equivalent**: Triceps extension

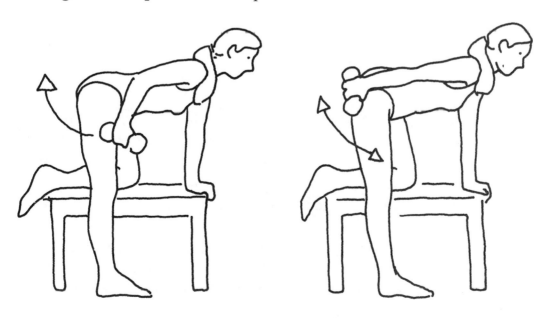

# Getting Your Doctor's Okay to Exercise

If you're just beginning an exercise program, show this plan to your doctor to make sure it's appropriate for you. If you have any of the following health conditions, you may need to be on a modified exercise program under your doctor's supervision:

- Heart disease or other heart condition
- High blood pressure
- Pregnancy
- History of breathing problems (including asthma)
- Chest pain during physical activity
- Bone or joint problems
- Diabetes
- Previous episodes of dizziness or loss of consciousness

# Your Weekly Exercise Plan

If you're new to exercise, you'll need to ease into your exercise routine—building up from a fifteen-minute to an hour's walk during your first few weeks, for example. This plan will help you build up your stamina while minimizing your risk of injury during the first six weeks. Each week, you'll increase and extend your activities until you're going full force during the sixth week and beyond.

If at any time you find you've increased your intensity beyond your fitness level, go back to your previous fitness routine until you feel it has become too easy. Then you can move on to the next week on the plan. By the same token, if week one feels too easy for your fitness level, skip ahead to a week where you feel comfortable. Remember: If you don't feel like you're working hard enough, you should be increasing the intensity or duration of your activity. For strength training, you should be increasing the poundage of the weights or number of sets.

As you'll see, the plan gives you one day off a week. You can take this day whenever you choose—perhaps on a particularly hectic day when you just can't squeeze in a workout.

All you need to do now is choose the aerobic activity you've decided to try, make a list of the equipment and clothing you'll need, and get moving! (Of course, don't forget to get your doctor's go-ahead before you begin.)

## WEEK ONE

**Sunday**
Warm-up 5 minutes
Stretch 5 minutes
Aerobic Activity 15–20 minutes
Stretch 5 minutes

**Monday**
Warm-up 5 minutes
Stretch 5 minutes
Strength Training Routine: 1 set of all exercises
   (8–12 reps)
Stretch 5 minutes

**Tuesday**
Warm-up 5 minutes
Stretch 5 minutes
Aerobic Activity 15–20 minutes
Stretch 5 minutes

**Wednesday**
Day Off

**Thursday**
Warm-up 5 minutes
Stretch 5 minutes
Strength Training Routine: 1 set of all exercises
   (8–12 reps)
Stretch 5 minutes
Day Off

**Friday**
Warm-up 5 minutes
Stretch 5 minutes
Aerobic Activity 15–20 minutes
Stretch 5 minutes

**Saturday**
Family Fun Day*

*Family Fun Days can be taken on any day of the week, although weekends are usually most convenient. Use this as an occasion to be active with your family or friends. Take a nature hike, go skating in the park, frolic in the waves at the beach. Go to the local Y and play a game of one-on-one basketball or get a game of volleyball going. Maybe you and your spouse always wanted to learn to horseback ride or take tae kwon do. Seize the day!

# WEEK TWO

**Sunday**
Warm-up 5 minutes
Stretch 5 minutes
Aerobic Activity 25 minutes
Stretch 5 minutes

**Monday**
Warm-up 5 minutes
Stretch 5 minutes
Strength Training Routine: 1 set of all exercises
    (12–15 reps)
Stretch 5 minutes

**Tuesday**
Warm-up 5 minutes
Stretch 5 minutes
Aerobic Activity 25 minutes
Stretch 5 minutes

**Wednesday**
Warm-up 5 minutes
Stretch 5 minutes
Strength Training Routine: 1 set of all exercises
    (12–15 reps)
Stretch 5 minutes

**Thursday**
Warm-up 5 minutes
Stretch 5 minutes
Aerobic Activity 30–35 minutes
Cool-down & Stretch 10 minutes

**Friday**
Warm-up 5 minutes
Stretch 5 minutes
Aerobic Activity 25 minutes
Stretch 5 minutes

**Saturday**
Family Fun Day

# WEEK THREE

**Sunday**
Warm-up 5 minutes
Stretch 5 minutes
Aerobic Activity 30–35 minutes
Cool-down & Stretch 10 minutes

**Monday**
Day Off

**Tuesday**
Warm-up 5 minutes
Stretch 5 minutes
Aerobic Activity 30–35 minutes
Cool-down & Stretch 10 minutes

**Wednesday**
Warm-up 5 minutes
Stretch 5 minutes
Strength Training Routine: 2 sets of all exercises
    (8 reps)
Stretch 5 minutes

**Thursday**
Warm-up 5 minutes
Stretch 5 minutes
Aerobic Activity 40 minutes
Cool-down & Stretch 10 minutes

**Friday**
Warm-up 5 minutes
Stretch 5 minutes
Strength Training Routine: 2 sets of all exercises
    (8 reps)
Stretch 5 minutes

**Saturday**
Family Fun Day

# WEEK FOUR

**Sunday**
Warm-up 5 minutes
Stretch 5 minutes
Aerobic Activity 40 minutes
Cool-down & Stretch 10 minutes

**Monday**
Warm-up 5 minutes
Stretch 5 minutes
Strength Training Routine: 2 sets of all exercises
    (12 reps)
Aerobic Activity 20 minutes
Cool-down & Stretch 10 minutes

**Tuesday**
Warm-up 5 minutes
Stretch 5 minutes
Aerobic Activity 40 minutes
Cool-down & Stretch 10 minutes

**Wednesday**
Day Off

**Thursday**
Warm-up 5 minutes
Stretch 5 minutes
Aerobic Activity 45–50 minutes
Cool-down & Stretch 10 minutes

**Friday**
Warm-up 5 minutes
Stretch 5 minutes
Strength Training Routine: 2 sets of all exercises
    (12 reps)
Aerobic Activity 20 minutes
Cool-down & Stretch 10 minutes

**Saturday**
Family Fun Day

# WEEK FIVE

**Sunday**
Warm-up 5 minutes
Stretch 5 minutes
Aerobic Activity 45–50 minutes
Cool-down & Stretch 10 minutes

**Monday**
Warm-up 5 minutes
Stretch 5 minutes
Strength Training Routine: 2 sets of all exercises
    (15 reps)
Aerobic Activity 25 minutes
Cool-down & Stretch 10 minutes

**Tuesday**
Warm-up 5 minutes
Stretch 5 minutes
Aerobic Activity 45–50 minutes
Cool-down & Stretch 10 minutes

**Wednesday**
Warm-up 5 minutes
Stretch 5 minutes
Strength Training Routine: 2 sets of all exercises
    (15 reps)
Aerobic Activity 25 minutes
Cool-down & Stretch 10 minutes

**Thursday**
Warm-up 5 minutes
Aerobic Activity 30 minutes
Cool-down & Stretch 10 minutes
Stretch 5 minutes
Strength Training Routine: 1 set (8 reps) at
    heavier weight and 1 set (12 reps) at regular
    weight

**Friday**
Day Off

**Saturday**
Family Fun Day

## WEEK SIX

**Sunday**
Day Off

**Monday**
Warm-up 5 minutes
Stretch 5 minutes
Aerobic Activity 50 minutes–1 hour
Cool-down & Stretch 10 minutes

**Tuesday**
Warm-up 5 minutes
Stretch 5 minutes
Aerobic Activity 30 minutes
Cool-down & Stretch 10 minutes
Strength Training Routine: 1 set (8 reps) at
    heavier weight and 1 set (12 reps) at regular
    weight

**Wednesday**
Warm-up 5 minutes
Stretch 5 minutes
Aerobic Activity 50 minutes–1 hour
Cool-down & Stretch 10 minutes

**Thursday**
Warm-up 5 minutes
Aerobic Activity 30 minutes
Stretch 5 minutes
Strength Training Routine: 1 set (8 reps) at
    heavier weight and 1 set (12 reps) at regular
    weight
Cool-down & Stretch 10 minutes

**Friday**
Warm-up 5 minutes
Stretch 5 minutes
Aerobic Activity 50 minutes–1 hour
Cool Down & Stretch 10 minutes

**Saturday**
Family Fun Day

You're off to a great start! Remember: It's important to choose exercises you enjoy doing. If you get bored, then you'll know it's time to vary your workouts, or look for a new activity altogether. Your body doesn't care how you get it moving, as long as you're working your heart and the rest of your muscles. Keep it up, and revel in the way you feel!

## Creating Your Personal Relaxation Plan

How many times have you used food to take the edge off a particularly trying day? When you have a hard time at work, it's easy enough—*too* easy—to lose yourself in a desk-drawer stash of chocolate chip cookies. After you've run twenty minutes late for every errand and appointment you had all day, kicking back in front of the TV and digging into a box of cookies can be an irresistible way to forget all the stress. But this quick-fix relief comes with a hefty price tag—unwanted pounds.

Exercise can be a great stress reliever, but it's all about *invigoration*; ideally, it should be offset with an equally important dose of *relaxation*. The Body•Mind•Life Makeover is designed to help you achieve that relaxation, giving you a kind of mini-vacation every single day—a small pocket of time to clear your mind and step away from the craziness of life.

Relaxation doesn't mean sinking into your couch and vegging out in front of the TV—a time when you may be kicking back, but your mind may well be worrying over the stresses of the day. True relaxation is the art of *letting go*. It's all about releasing tension from your muscles and sweeping away troubling thoughts. And in order to achieve complete relaxation, both mind and body must be free of that tension.

## Bad Habits—and How to Ban Them

It's one of life's great lessons: We are our own caretakers—or, to put it another way, we're our own mothers. If we don't take care of ourselves, it won't get done. No one can be a good parent if they spend all their time making excuses, saying "Oh, I'm too busy working," or "I can't take care of you—I've got friends who need me." Likewise, if you want to lead the happiest life, the best thing you can do is stop making excuses and start turning your attention to taking care of yourself.

Here's one thing I've learned about myself: Whenever I catch myself falling into a little self-destructive pattern—taking on everyone else's problems as my own, trying to mediate relatives' holiday problems over the phone from 2,000 miles away—I feel like going straight to the refrigerator for a dose of comfort food. I used to be the same way about smoking. Before I quit, whenever I was taking on too much stress I'd reach for a cigarette; sometimes I'd have a cigarette in one hand and a lit match in the other before I realized what I was doing.

I've banished my old stress-binge eating habits just the same way I quit smoking: Every time I got one of those anxious "hunger" pangs, I'd take a deep breath and remove myself from the situation to focus on exactly what I was feeling. Usually it only takes five or ten minutes of concentration before your equilibrium settles back into place. And so what if you feel like crying or kicking something? Everyone feels that way every now and then; if you're not alone, head for a bathroom or take a walk around the block. It's a nice way to sneak a little meditation—a little private time—into your own life. Try making this a practice, and if you can do it for twenty-one days, the way I did, you'll find you've kicked the bad-eating habit.

## Good Habits—and How to Make Them

We are creatures of habit, but what many people never realize is that we can *choose* our habits. Just as we owe it to ourselves to drop our bad habits, it's in our best interest to cultivate the positive habits that make up a healthy lifestyle.

Here's one: *Breathe.* The most important thing we do in life is breathing, but most of us never give it a second thought. Air is our number one food; it comes before water, before eatables, before anything. I make it a point to take deep breaths all day long, because the body runs on oxygen—the oxygen we draw from the air into our lungs, which then enriches the blood and fuels the rest of our bodily functions. Exercise will help you breathe deeply, but even when you're just sitting at your desk quietly, every so often pull in a nice, long breath of air. It'll do you good.

Here's another: *Drink water.* Most of us don't get as much as we need.

When I'm in the city, I buy it bottled or put it through a water-purification system; when I'm out west I drink well water that I've filtered to eliminate lead and other impurities. I keep water bottles with me wherever I go: by my desk, in the car, by the TV—in every room in the house, in fact. Since I started upping my water intake (I make it a point to have at least six big glasses a day, always trying for eight), I find that everything works better—especially my plumbing. And here's another discovery I made: It's a wonder for wrinkles! It turns out moisturizing from the *inside* is even more important than applying oils or creams on the outside.

The all-important third habit: *Eat right*. Slim•Fast makes it easy with two shakes or meal bars a day, but they didn't come up with the phrase "sensible dinner" for nothing. It's important to eat as many fresh foods, and as few processed foods, as possible. Reduce your intake of heavy meats, and increase your vegetables and fruits to compensate. It's much easier to find organic foods (and great-tasting organic food at that!) anywhere in the country than it used to be, and many more people every year are introducing tofu and other soy dishes into their diets. I also make it a point to cook with olive oil, which is the healthiest variety, and to have good raw vegetables on hand for snacking all day long. (And when I get that creeping lust just to be *around* food, I often find it great to take some time to fix a big bowl of tabouleh—a wonderful melange of vegetables and grains, which takes plenty of time in the chopping and can stay fresh in the fridge for days. It's the perfect snack food.)

And, personally, I do believe in taking *vitamins and minerals* every day. Every morning, along with my Slim•Fast, I take vitamin C and beta-carotene; at lunch I take vitamin E and selenium, along with a calcium-magnesium combination and one aspirin (because my family has a history of heart disease). There are a lot of other supplements on the market, of course, and there seem to be more cropping up all the time. But these are my staples, the ones I've been taking every day for years.

# Eliciting the Relaxation Response

To make over your mind and mental outlook, the plan will teach you how to elicit "the relaxation response"—a term coined by relaxation researcher Herbert Benson, M.D., author of *Timeless Healing* and president of the Mind/Body Medical Institute at Harvard's Beth Israel Deaconess Medical Center. You'll actually be calming all your body's systems. You'll lower your blood pressure and decrease your heart rate and breathing rate. Research also suggests that eliciting the relaxation response boosts your brain's production of the feel-good chemicals serotonin and endorphins, which will increase your sense of calm and happiness.

In over two decades of research, Benson and his colleagues have determined that getting your body into a relaxed state can have a host of health benefits, from lowering your risk of heart disease to curing insomnia to restoring a happier outlook to your life. Eliciting the relaxation response has another added benefit: It can actually help reduce your craving for sweets by regulating the release of cortisol, a stress hormone that can wreak havoc with blood sugar levels and convince your body it needs more sugar.

Given all these obvious advantages, it's important to learn to relax on demand—even if it means actively ignoring the source of your stress. Choose one of the relaxation techniques below (or try a different technique each day); *give yourself fifteen to twenty minutes a day to get your body into a completely relaxed state.* Skip that mediocre sitcom between your two favorite shows, or close your door during your coffee break at work. Just be sure to choose a time of day when you can unplug the phone and be free of any distractions.

# Your Getaway Options

**The traditional way:** Dr. Benson has developed and tested this method of eliciting the relaxation response: First, sit comfortably and pick a focus word or short phrase that's meaningful to you. Close your eyes and relax your muscles. Now, breathe slowly and naturally, repeating your focus word or phrase silently as you exhale.

Throughout, assume a passive attitude. Don't worry about whether you're performing the technique correctly. When other thoughts come to mind, simply let them pass without pondering them. Gently return to your repetition. Continue for fifteen to twenty minutes. You may open your eyes to check the time, but don't use an alarm—it'll only disrupt your relaxation. When you finish, sit quietly for a minute or so, at first with your eyes closed and then with your eyes open. Remain seated for one or two minutes before standing.

**Progressive muscle relaxation:** Sit in a comfortable chair with back and head support, or lie on a lightly cushioned mat on the floor. (A bed is too soft and will make you more likely to fall asleep.) Tense each of your muscles one at a time; inhale and slowly exhale as you release the tension from your muscles. Begin with your face by wrinkling your forehead and shutting your eyes as tight as you can. Exhale and release. Then tense your neck and shoulders by drawing your shoulders up into a shrug. Exhale and release. Work your way down to your arms and hands, pressing your palms together with your elbows pointing outward and push as hard as you can. Exhale and release. Contract your stomach. Exhale and release. Arch your back and release. Now tense your hips and buttocks, pressing your legs and heels against the surface beneath you. Exhale and release. Point and flex your toes and release.

Now tense all your muscles at once. Then take a deep breath, hold it, and exhale slowly as you relax the muscles, letting go of the tension. Feel your body at rest and enjoy this state of relaxation for several minutes. When you're first learning this technique, you may want to create a tape recording, reading slowly through the above instructions. You can play the recording while you're relaxing your muscles to make sure you don't skip any of the muscle groups.

**Meditation:** The focused awareness that comes with meditation can let you appreciate the interconnectedness of all living things. Sit comfortably in an upright position with your head, neck, and back erect but not stiff. You can sit in a straight-backed chair or cross-legged on the floor. Choose a single object of focus like your breathing or a portion of a prayer. Concentrate on the qualities of that object, the sounds, sensations, and thoughts, as they enter into your awareness.

You can also practice meditation in a natural setting such as an outdoor garden, or while sitting by a window. Watch the sun set, the clouds drift, or the stars twinkle, and focus on the air flowing in and out of your body as you breathe. Appreciating the beauty of nature allows you to transcend your own problems and reminds you of how vast the world really is.

**Strike a pose:** Yoga can help increase your sense of serenity. What's more, you'll be improving your body tone and flexibility at the same time. You should move through the various poses slowly and mindfully to get the benefit of relaxation. You can learn yoga by taking a class (which is probably the best method, since an instructor can correct your form) or through a book or video.

For information on classes in your area, check out http://www.yogafinder.com. You can try a practice class on the Internet by logging onto www.yogaclass.com. Good yoga books include *20-Minute Yoga Workouts* by Alice Christensen (Fawcett Books, 1995) and *Light on Yoga: Yoga Dipika* by B. K. S. Iyengar and Yehudi Menuhin (Shocken Books, 1995). Good yoga videos include *Yoga for Meditators* with John Friend; *Living Yoga AM/PM Practice* with Rodney Yee and Patricia Waldern; and *Yoga: Mind and Body* with Eric Shiffman and Ali MacGraw.

**Relaxation quickie:** When you feel your tension rising, you may not be in a position to take a twenty-minute relaxation break. In these situations, you can use this quick and effective technique described by Dr. Christian Northrup: Press your hand over your heart and close your eyes. While breathing deeply, recall someone or something you love completely and unconditionally. Feel that loving feeling for a minute or so. Open your eyes and take a deep breath. It'll help you remember what life is really all about.

Now that you've got the basics of the Slim•Fast Body•Mind•Life Makeover, you're ready to put it all together and begin living a new life. At times, you'll find you need to work hard to maintain your healthy habits. Just remember how good you feel and how great you've already begun to look as a result of your new life. Reward yourself once in a while with a new outfit or a fun night out on the town. In fact, that's what the next chapter is all about— celebrating your new life. You'll see that you can still eat out and enjoy parties while maintaining your healthy lifestyle. It's time to have your cake and eat it, too!

# 8

---

# CELEBRATE
# YOUR NEW LIFE!

As you plan and plot your meals, track your exercise, and pencil in your relaxation efforts, remember the most important element of the Slim•Fast Makeover: having fun. Fun is often the forgotten factor. After all, most diets put you through a type of boot camp: You deprive yourself until you reach your ultimate weight-loss goal—and then you're so hard up for fun that you can hardly be blamed for going overboard to make up for all those weeks of deprivation.

The Body•Mind•Life Makeover is all about getting pleasure in your life. The Slim•Fast products taste like milk shakes, fruit smoothies, and chocolate bars for one reason: so you'll enjoy them. Eating should always be a pleasurable experience. You may be controlling the amount of food you put in your mouth, but you should still be able to savor every mouthful. By the same token, your fitness activities should be fun and leave you feeling invigorated. Your relaxation practices should help you tap into the joy that comes with being alive and experiencing the simple pleasures of the world around you.

So if you've gotten this far into the plan, your life should already have become more enjoyable, filled with good food, invigorating exercise, and the excitement that comes from improving your life. Still, you may be wondering about some aspects of everyday life that might seem hard to reconcile with all your plans: What about my favorite restaurants? What about the office Christmas party? How will I make it through my family reunion without overindulging?

But there's no need to worry. You can live your normal social life without worrying about sacrificing your weight-loss efforts. All you need are some strategies for dealing with these situations.

You can absolutely eat out at good restaurants and live through a brush with a party buffet, as long as you make smart selections. Just think before you read. You can even eat a little fast food when you're off on a vacation road trip. The key is moderation. Just use common sense: Restrict your dining-out plans to once a week instead of picking up takeout four or five nights a week. Give yourself the green light to do anything you really want to do, but know when to flash the red light—stop before you feel too full. If you'll take the time to develop sensible strategies for navigating those tempting pitfalls, you'll have the satisfaction of making your own decisions about what goes into your body and how you feel every week.

Celebrating your new life also means finding pleasure in so much more than just food. For many of us food is a main source of pleasure, and that's fine—but it shouldn't be the *principal* source of comfort or solace. With your new body and new life, you'll find other outlets for pleasure and fun. Need to get some new clothes to fit your new body size? Be a little carefree and pick up a high-fashion blouse you normally wouldn't buy or a suit in a can't-miss color. Even a new scarf or different hairstyle can give you a new look to go with your new body and your new attitude. As part of your transformation, you may even find yourself feeling sexier; after all, your sex drive is a barometer of your overall health, and being in shape can make things easier in the bedroom on any number of levels—from physical stamina to confidence. Not a bad bonus, right?

Here are a few smart strategies to keep in mind as you venture out in the world.

## Smart Strategy 1: Map Out a Plan When Going to a Restaurant

Consider this: Women who eat out more than five times a week consume an average of 2,057 calories per day, compared to 1,769 calories for women who eat out less frequently. That adds up to a whopping weight gain of two pounds per month. Women who eat out also have a much higher fat intake—35 percent of their total daily calories, which is far above the recommended level of less than 30 percent. Some restaurant entrées contain enough fat and calories to cover an entire day's worth of meals. And that doesn't even include the bread, appetizer, or dessert! In recent years, restaurant portions have ballooned two or three times in size as restaurants compete for customers. "More is better" is their motto, and Americans have grown fatter as a result.

Eating out *can* throw a wrench into your weight-loss efforts, if you're not careful about what you put in your mouth. Still, there's no reason to forsake this pleasure for the good of your waistline. Eat out once or twice a week at most, and follow these rules to navigate the minefield of temptations:

**Analyze your own eating personality.** If you tend to go overboard when you go to a restaurant famished, try eating a light snack beforehand. A Slim•Fast snack bar or a piece of fruit with a small piece of cheese should keep hunger at bay, so you won't be as tempted to scarf down three rolls before your appetizer. On the other hand, if you know you can't restrict yourself when eating out, stick with much lighter meals earlier in the day. (If you have a Slim•Fast shake for both breakfast and lunch, you should feel just right for a healthy dinner.)

**Beware of the bread basket**. Tell your waiter to forgo the bread if the sight or scent of it is too tempting. If you still can't resist, take one piece (without butter) and divide it into three parts. Eat the first before you order, the second while waiting for the meal, and the third with your meal (with luck you won't even be tempted by then). This kind of portion control is a good strategy for any eating situation.

**Order from the appetizer/salad section of the menu**. Treating an appetizer as an entrée is a good way to save on calories, since appetizers tend to come in smaller portions. A soup and side salad can also make a filling meal, without the added calories and fat. But beware: Salads also sometimes come entrée-size, huge enough to feed two people. A plate filled with plain fresh vegetables won't contain many calories—but add some dressing, avocado, cheese, fish, or chicken to the mix and you've got a calorie-packed meal. If there's a huge salad you're dying to have, split it with your dining partner or ask for a side-salad portion.

**Dine à la carte.** You may be inclined to order a full meal—appetizer, dessert, and all—if it costs less than the sum of its parts. But this plan only sets you up to eat more. Don't force down a dessert just because it's included—especially if you aren't really hungry.

**Get the dressing on the side.** Many restaurants still don't offer fat-free dressings, or you may have a hankering for the real thing. Trouble is, salad dressings often get poured on in such quantities that your salad ends up being as fattening as a huge steak. Remember to control your calorie and fat intake by having it served on the side.

**Watch for hidden calories.** Many meals are loaded with calories, added in subtle ways. Oils are often added to tomato sauces; rich gravies or cream sauces are slathered over meats and vegetables. A low-fat filet of fish can be turned into a vehicle for fat by being breaded and fried. In general, the plainer the food, the better. Anything grilled or broiled, with a light sprinkling of spices, tends to be lower in calories than something bathed in a thicker sauce. Another surprising source of hidden calories: fresh fruit shakes, which often have added sugar. Consider these a dessert: They can contain as many calories as a slice of cake.

**Mind the alcohol.** Alcohol is loaded with calories, and it's easy to consume more than you want while you're in the social spirit. Stick to one glass of wine or beer with dinner, or a dessert aperitif. Remember, an 8-ounce beer, a 3½-ounce glass of wine, and a shot of liquor each contain about 100 calories; fruity tropical drinks can contain 300 or more.

**Make dessert conditional:** Before you order dessert, ask yourself two questions: Am I really still hungry? and Is this in my calorie budget for the day? Some low-calorie, healthy dessert options: fresh raspberries sprinkled on a small scoop of sorbet, or strawberries topped with a tiny squirt of whipped cream.

**Engage your partner**: Try to eat out with someone who will help you keep your temptations in check. The two of you can decide in advance what to order, before your restraint is weakened. Your partner can keep the breadbasket in a safe place, and refrain from pushing drinks or dessert.

**Let yourself off the hook**: If you eat more than you planned, don't consider it a catastrophe. Remember, it's unrealistic to think you'll never overeat. What you don't want to do is quit your weight-loss efforts because you think you've blown it. Keep the event in perspective and resolve to make a better go of it next time.

## Smart Strategy 2: With Fast Food, Think Salads and Child-Size Portions

You don't necessarily need to avoid fast-food establishments altogether. By popular demand, fast-food restaurants have evolved to include healthier options. Their chicken dishes can be lower in fat and calories than beef dishes—as long as you choose broiled or grilled dishes instead of fried chicken or nuggets. Healthier oils are being used to cook french fries in some places, though they're still loaded with the same amount of fat and calories. If you choose selectively, it is possible to walk into a fast-food restaurant and escape with a reasonable meal.

**Hit the salad bar**: Salad bars can be low-calorie or extremely high-calorie experiences, depending on what you choose. Pile your plate high with plain fresh vegetables; skip anything floating in oils or drenched in mayonnaise. Fat-free dressings are great, or just take a tiny drizzle of your favorite regular dressing. Another low-calorie option: Squeeze on some fresh lemon juice and a splash of balsamic vinegar.

**Stay away from the breaded and fried**: Anything that's covered in batter, grease, or a globby "special sauce" is bound to be loaded with fat and calories. Healthy low-fat options include a skinless grilled chicken breast sandwich

# What's Good on the Menu?

It can be difficult to tell the nutritious from the unhealthy on restaurant menus. Here's a guide to some lighter options and high-fat pitfalls, based on a series of nutritional analyses of restaurant foods conducted by the Center for Science in the Public Interest. "Best" choices have less than 30 grams of fat, a generous meal's worth for an active, medium-size person. "Worst" have up to 100 grams of fat.

## Fast Food

Best Choices
> Grilled chicken sandwich
> Roast beef sandwich
> Single hamburger
> Salad with light vinaigrette

Worst
> Double cheeseburger
> French fries
> Onion rings

*Tips:* Order sandwiches without mayo or "special sauce." Avoid deep-fried items like fish filets, chicken nuggets, and french fries.

## Italian

Best Choices
> Pasta with red or white sauce
> Spaghetti with marinara or tomato-and-meat sauce

Worst Choices
> Eggplant parmigiana
> Fettuccine Alfredo
> Lasagna

*Tips:* Stick with plain bread instead of garlic bread made with butter or oil. Ask for the waiter's help in avoiding cream- or egg-based sauces.

# Chinese

Best

 Hot-and-sour soup

 Stir-fried vegetables

 Grilled chicken

 Wonton soup

Worst Choices

 Crispy chicken

 Kung pao chicken

*Tips:* Share a stir-fry; mix your dish with a helping of steamed rice. Ask for vegetables steamed or stir-fried with less oil. Order moo shu vegetables instead of a meat-based dish. Avoid fried rice, breaded dishes, and items loaded with nuts.

# Sandwiches

Best Choices

 Roast beef

 Turkey

Worst Choices

 Tuna salad

 Reuben

 Submarine

*Tips:* Ask for mustard; hold the mayo and cheese. See if turkey-bologna or turkey-pastrami is available.

# Mexican

Best Choices

        Bean burrito (no cheese)

        Chicken fajitas

Worst Choices

        Beef chimichanga

        Chile relleno

        Quesadilla

        Refried beans

*Tips:* Choose soft tortillas with fresh salsa, not guacamole. Special-order fish or chicken. Ask for beans made without lard or fat.

# Seafood

Best Choices

        Broiled bass, halibut, or snapper

        Grilled salmon

Worst Choices

        Fried seafood platter

        Blackened catfish

*Tips:* Order fish broiled, baked, grilled, or steamed—not pan-fried or sautéed. Ask for lemon instead of tartar sauce. Avoid creamy or buttery sauces.

topped with chopped vegetables, a plain broiled fish, or a grilled vegetable burger. Try a plain baked potato or rice instead of fries.

**Stick with child-size portions:** If you must order fries, get the small size. If you have a hankering for a hamburger, order a child-size meal. Reducing portion sizes will help keep calories and fat under control.

**Forgo regular soft drinks:** Go for diet sodas rather than regular versions, which are loaded with sugar and empty calories. And stay away from milkshakes, which can have more calories and fat than your main course.

# Smart Strategy 3: Party! (with Restraint)

Parties can be major pitfalls when you're trying to lose weight, since you have no control over what is served. Even the seemingly harmless handfuls of nibbles you grab here and there from tables and hors d'oeuvre trays can really add up. Still, you don't need to skip parties altogether. Just go with a game plan like this one.

**Don't arrive hungry.** Take the edge off hunger before you leave home by eating something light but satisfying, like a handful of pretzels or a Slim•Fast snack bar.

**Allow yourself a little splurge.** Denying yourself all the temptations you see at parties could set you up for an eating binge when you get home. When you first arrive, survey the scene and see which food looks the most tempting. Allow yourself that piece of chocolate fudge or slice of cheesecake, but don't try everything. If you want to sample a few things, stick with modest portions and smaller bites. You'll satisfy your curiosity without packing in the calories.

**Avoid mindless eating.** This is hard to do at a party when you're chattering away and not really paying attention to what you're putting in your mouth. Try to establish particular eating times, rather than eating throughout the party. Do one modest round of the finger foods and one of the desserts. Avoid going back for seconds.

**Keep in mind that alcohol's calories count.** A 12-ounce beer and 7-ounce glass of wine each contain 150 calories. A shot of 90-proof whiskey contains 110 calories. Having two or three drinks at a party can send your daily calorie count spinning out of control. If you're going to indulge in alcohol, stick with lower-calorie foods. Better yet, have just one drink and then stick with seltzer and a twist of lime.

**Make some smart food substitutions.** Use the chart below as a guide.

| Instead of . . . | Choose . . . |
|---|---|
| 3 sugar cookies (265 cal, 9 g fat) | 3 gingersnaps (100 cal, 6 g fat) |
| 1 ounce potato chips (150 cal, 10 g fat) | 1 ounce pretzels (100 cal, 1 g fat) |
| 1 ounce chocolate fudge with nuts (120 cal, 5 g fat) | 2 chocolate-covered strawberries (40 cal, 2 g fat) |
| 1 mini-quiche (150 cal, 12 g fat) | 2 medium spinach-stuffed mushrooms (44 cal, 1 g fat) |

# Smart Strategy 4: Use a Lapse to Help Get You Back on Track

In the name of having a little fun, you may find you want to let the rules slide from time to time. Perhaps you used your two-week cruise as a vacation from your makeover plan. Or maybe you've been cheating a little more each day. The fact is, everyone cheats from time to time—including people who are successful at maintaining a weight loss. The key is in how you deal with these lapses—whether you throw in the towel or get yourself back on track. Once you realize you've fallen off the wagon, follow these seven steps developed by G. Alan Marlatt, Ph.D., a psychologist from the University of Washington in Seattle.

**Step 1: Stop, look, and listen.** A lapse is a signal of impending danger, like flashing lights at a train crossing. Stop a moment—especially if the lapse is still in progress—and examine the situation. Can you afford this lapse? Consider removing yourself to a safe situation away from the temptations to avoid overindulging.

**Step 2: Stay calm.** If you get anxious or blame yourself for the lapse, you may conclude that you're a hopeless binge eater with no control. Try to separate yourself from the situation and realize what an objective observer would—that one lapse doesn't make your efforts a failure.

**Step 3: Renew your weight-loss vows.** Take a minute to remind yourself of how far you've come and how sad it would be if one lapse canceled out all your work. Remind yourself of your goals and renew the vows you made when you began the program.

**Step 4: Analyze the lapse situation.** Instead of blaming yourself for letting go, use the situation to learn what places you at risk. Do certain feelings trigger overeating? Does the presence of food or other activities tempt you consistently? Have you done anything to defend against the urge? Did it work? Why or why not? What would you do differently in the future?

**Step 5: Take charge immediately.** Leap into action; waiting is just another excuse for letting go. Leave the house, throw the remaining food into the garbage, or do whatever works for you. You might try to schedule a workout and plan your next day's meals to get yourself back on track.

**Step 6: Make Slim•Fast your next meal.** This can be a great way to get back on track.

**Step 7: Ask for help.** Partners, friends, co-workers, and others can be a real source of support, providing perspective and offering the encouragement you may need.


# Smart Strategy 5: Live Your Life with Style

Style has nothing to do with body size, and it isn't about settling for clothes that "just fit," either. Your personal style should feature clothes that fit your life and flatter your body. If you're trying to lose weight—whether it's 15, 25, or 50 pounds or more—you'll certainly need to consider your changing body in the choices you make. You also need to consider the type of life you lead: whether you work in a corporate or a casual environment, what you do in your leisure time, what climate you live in. On top of this, you should consider your own personal style preferences (are you classic or trendy? quiet or outgoing?) and taste in color. When all of these things come together, your own individual style begins to emerge. This style will reflect the new you that you've become.

Nearly half of all American women currently fit in the size range 14 to 24, now known as the "plus size" category. Designers and manufacturers have finally realized that shapeless tent dresses just don't cut it anymore for large-size women. These women want the four Fs: fit, function, and figure-flattery. Clothes that provide ample coverage while streamlining your shape can do wonders for your self-confidence while you're trying to lose weight. Finding clothes that move smoothly from one point on the scale to the next—as well as from day to night and season to season—can help you maintain your sense of style and feel good about the way you look.

**Highlight what you like and minimize what you don't.** You want to bring out your body's best features. If you want to play up your great legs while minimizing your stomach, choose a stitched-down pleat-front skirt that falls above the knee. Long sleeves can cover fuller arms, while a halter-cut blouse flatters a large bust and emphasizes shoulders. If you've got a large derriere, wear an A-line or flared skirt (not pleated or form-fitting) and loose-fitting pants.

**Shop before you drop.** Don't wait until you get to your goal weight before buying new clothes. Purchasing a great-where-you-are wardrobe basic, like a classic blue men's shirt, tells you that you deserve to look good now, though you can still wear it as you transition from one size down to a lower one. Also, the better you feel about yourself in clothes, the more motivated you'll be to move into a smaller size.

**Stay in touch with your body.** Knowing your good and not-so-good points will clue you in to dressing for slimming success. Follow this color adage: Dark recedes and light reflects. Dark colors should stay below the hips, light colors above. To maximize height and slenderness, wear all one color. You should also take note of where you gain and lose weight first. When choosing an outfit, give yourself a little extra room in these areas to allow for a 2- or 3-pound weight fluctuation.

**Try a slenderizer.** If you're working out hard, but not getting the results as quickly as you'd like, you can still flatten your stomach and smooth out your hips with the new body slenderizers. Updated and more comfortable versions of the traditional girdle, they're made from body-sleeking Spandex and can be found in most women's lingerie departments.

**Build a transitional wardrobe.** While you're losing weight, you should have a core group of basics you can easily interchange with other separates. Look through your closet to determine which separates you need. All seven pieces mix and match with each other, especially if you stick mainly with neutral colors like gray, black, taupe, white, or brown.

*Long jacket:* Go for a gently fitted style that subtly defines your waist in a fingertip length to provide ample coverage of your hips and derriere.

*Classic white shirt:* A great lightweight layering piece. A men's style will give you an oversized effect. Can be worn under a suit, over a T-shirt and leggings, knotted at the waist with a skirt or pants, or even over a bathing suit.

*Tunic-length sweater:* Works like the long jacket for a more casual look. Use with both long and short hemlines.

*Classic crew-neck T-shirt:* Good for layering without the bulk.

*Straight or A-line skirt:* A strong vertical line visually adds height to your frame while minimizing width.

*Straight or full-leg trousers:* Straight up-and-down slims as it hides pounds.

*Leggings:* Sleek body-hugging leggings will make you look slimmer than bulky jeans. Pair them with a long shirt or jacket to cover areas you don't want to emphasize.

Fattening styles to avoid:

Big floral patterns
Bold prints
Big patch pockets
Oversize buttons, touches, and trims
Horizontal patterns
Trouser cuffs
Bulky fabrics
Big wide belts
Oversize, heavy pocketbooks
Head-hugging hats

What's most important is that you find the time to kick back and break free from the daily grind. Socializing with friends and having a blast with your family can renew your spirit and give you a fresh outlook on life. The thing to keep in mind is, living healthy and having fun don't need to be mutually exclusive. Both are essential to the success of your makeover plan. In fact, once you're under way you may even find yourself eager to share your new life with others. That's what the next chapter is all about.

# 9

# ENTERTAINING
# THE SLIM•FAST WAY

**P**lanning a family dinner for the holidays or a casual get-together for friends always sounds great in theory—that is, until you start the shopping and the cooking. Preparations can gobble up time you would normally spend exercising or relaxing. You may also be nervous about having leftover high-fat goodies in the house after your guests leave. The good news is, you can have people over for an enjoyable, delicious meal without sacrificing your good health habits. Even better, no one will think they're eating "diet" food. In fact, you'll probably find friends and relatives asking for your recipes.

The menus that follow are designed to give you a balanced meal—complete with low-fat protein, carbohydrates, and plenty of fruits and vegetables—that you can prepare for a small group. They represent one perfect way to share your new life with your friends and extended family. You'll also encounter some helpful hints to help you stay on the right track. Who says planning a party can't be as much fun as attending one?

## Serving Light at a Party

So you're planning a little gathering with thirty or so of your closest friends. Or maybe it's your turn to host the family reunion. Whatever the occasion, you can keep the menu light and still dazzle your guests. Here's how:

**Serve buffet-style**. It's faster, simpler, and easier on you—and it lets your guests choose their own portion sizes. No one will feel pressured to take more or less than they want.

**Don't call it "health food."** Most people think of "health food" as tasteless and bland. Don't feel compelled to explain—just serve and wait for the compliments.

**Go for volume**. A healthy meal doesn't have to mean a small portion. If you watch the fat content and provide a wide variety of vegetables, fruits, and grains, even hearty eaters won't feel deprived.

**Impress with exotic finds**. A salad with unusual greens and flower petals can delight just as much as a Cornish game hen—with far fewer calories.

**Garnish, garnish, garnish**. Try edible flowers, prettily carved fruits and vegetables, curly purple kale leaves, or fresh herbs or vines to liven up your presentation; you can even create an edible centerpiece to bring your table to life.

# Parties with an Active Theme

Who says parties have to be all about food? Why not have a theme party that gets you and your guests active? Here are some suggestions.

**Summer Solstice Party**: Celebrate the coming of summer by trying some informal summer sports at your backyard barbecue. Set up a badminton net. Break out the croquet set. Grab a basketball and divide into teams for a friendly game.

**Scavenger Hunt**: What better way to meet your neighbors than by having a scavenger hunt? Give your guests lists of wacky things they have to find and send them walking throughout your neighborhood or a nearby park.

**Beach Party**: Bring a cooler stocked with sandwiches, fruit, and cold drinks, and have a party on the beach. Play a little beach volleyball or paddleball. Jump and ride the waves. Go for a group walk.

**Bike to a Picnic Party**: Get a few friends together and strap a picnic basket to the back of your bike. Bike over to a secluded spot and spread your blanket.

Think of your social gatherings as a chance to celebrate life. Your guests don't need to leave feeling stuffed in order to have a good time. By preparing meals that work the Slim•Fast way, you'll be giving your guests a dose of healthy living, energy, and vitality. Who says good health and good times can't go hand in hand?

# Recipes for Entertaining

## HOLIDAY BRUNCH

**Caesar Salad (page 315)**
**Dilly Vegetable Sauté**
**Chicken Scaloppini Limone**
**Spinach Manicotti**
**Cinnamon–Spiced Peaches with Vanilla Frozen Yogurt**

## Dilly Vegetable Sauté

*Total preparation time: 25 minutes*

Nonstick cooking spray
2 teaspoons olive oil
1 medium yellow onion, peeled and diced
1 clove garlic, peeled and minced
1 pound carrots, tops and bottoms removed, peeled, halved, then cut into
    1-inch diagonal pieces
1 pound green beans, stringed and washed
1 tablespoon chopped fresh dill
½ pound pea pods, trimmed and washed

1.  Lightly coat a large nonstick skillet or wok with cooking spray, add oil, and heat over medium-high flame. Add onions and garlic and sauté, turning occasionally, until onions soften, 5 minutes.
2.  Add carrots and turn heat to medium. Cover and cook 5 to 7 minutes, until carrots begin to soften. Add beans, cover, and cook another 5 minutes, turning frequently. Add dill and pea pods, and continue to cook uncovered, turning frequently, until pea pods are soft but still bright green, 2 to 3 minutes. Transfer to a platter and serve.

SERVES 8

# Chicken Scaloppini Limone

*Total preparation time: 25 minutes*

1¾ pounds boneless, skinless chicken breasts
½ cup unbleached white flour
Nonstick cooking spray
1 tablespoon olive oil
¼ cup fresh lemon juice
⅓ cup chopped fresh parsley
1 pound mushrooms, ends trimmed, washed, and sliced
1 lemon, thinly sliced

1.  Place chicken breasts between two pieces of wax paper and pound with meat mallet or rolling pin until thin.
2.  Place flour on a plate. Dip chicken in flour, coating on both sides, and place on large plate.
3.  Lightly coat a large nonstick skillet with cooking spray and add oil over medium-high flame. Add lemon juice and chicken and sauté, turning frequently, until cooked and no longer pink inside, 6 to 7 minutes. Remove from pan with a slotted spoon and set aside.
4.  Add parsley and mushrooms to pan and sauté, turning occasionally, until

mushrooms are soft, 4 to 5 minutes. Spoon sauce over chicken, garnish with lemon slices, and serve.

SERVES 8

# Spinach Manicotti

*Total preparation time: 55 minutes*

¾ cup shredded part-skim mozzarella cheese
1½ cups fat-free ricotta cheese
1½ cups low-fat (1%) cottage cheese
¼ cup grated fresh Romano cheese
½ teaspoon dried Italian seasoning
One 10-ounce box frozen chopped spinach, thawed, drained, and squeezed dry
1 egg white
1 clove garlic, peeled and minced
One 8-ounce box uncooked manicotti shells
Nonstick cooking spray
One 26-ounce jar low-fat prepared tomato sauce

1. Preheat oven to 350°F. Set a large covered pot of water to boil.
2. In a large bowl, combine ½ cup of the mozzarella with all of the ricotta, cottage cheese, Romano, Italian seasoning, spinach, egg white, and garlic. Stir well and set aside.
3. Meanwhile, cook manicotti according to package directions, omitting salt and fat; do not overcook. Drain and rinse under cold water.
4. Lightly coat a 13 x 9-inch baking dish with cooking spray. Place manicotti in baking dish, spoon cheese mixture evenly into cooked pasta, and top with tomato sauce.
5. Bake, uncovered, in 350°F oven 25 minutes. Sprinkle with the remaining ¼ cup mozzarella cheese and bake 10 more minutes, or until cheese melts.

SERVES 8

# Cinnamon-Spiced Peaches with Vanilla Frozen Yogurt

*Total preparation time: 15 minutes*

6 large peaches, washed, pitted, and thinly sliced

½ cup craisins (dried, sweetened cranberries)

½ cup peach nectar

1 tablespoon dark brown sugar

½ teaspoon ground cinnamon

1 quart frozen vanilla nonfat yogurt

In a large covered saucepan, combine peaches with craisins, peach nectar, sugar, and cinnamon. Cook over medium heat 10 minutes, stirring occasionally. Serve over frozen yogurt.

SERVES 8

## NUTRITIONAL INFORMATION PER SERVING

|  | Calories | Protein | Carbohydrate | Fat | Fiber | Sodium | Cholesterol | Calcium |
|---|---|---|---|---|---|---|---|---|
| **Caesar salad** | 88 | 5 g | 14 g | 2 g (20%) | 2 g | 361 mg | 4 mg | 110 mg |
| **Dilly Vegetable Sauté** | 70 | 2.5 g | 13 g | 1.5 g (17%) | 4 g | 27 mg | 0 mg | 58 mg |
| **Chicken Scaloppini Limone** | 301 | 38.5 g | 9 g | 11 g (35%) | 1 g | 91 mg | 103 mg | 25 mg |
| **Spinach Manicotti** | 299 | 21 g | 37 g | 7 g (22%) | 4 g | 642 mg | 25 mg | 339 mg |
| **Cinnamon-Spiced Peaches with Vanilla Frozen Yogurt** | 169 | 4.5 g | 38.5 g | 0.5 g (1%) | 2 g | 82 mg | 0 mg | 108 mg |

## MEMORIAL DAY PICNIC

**Chicken Bowtie Salad**
**Garden Salad**
**Marinated Green Bean and Tomato Salad**
**Herbed Yogurt Cheese**
**Triple Berry Fruit Salad**

# Chicken Bowtie Salad

*Total preparation time: 1 hour*

3½ pounds boneless, skinless chicken breasts
1 pound bowtie pasta
Two 10-ounce boxes frozen peas, thawed
6 carrots, tops and bottoms removed, peeled, and cut into ¼-inch slices
3 stalks celery, trimmed, washed, and finely diced
2 large red peppers, washed, cored, seeded, and diced
¼ cup extra-virgin olive oil
¼ cup fresh lemon juice
1 cup fat-free mayonnaise
½ cup finely chopped fresh parsley
1 tablespoon Dijon-style mustard
1 tablespoon grated lemon rind, yellow part only (no white pith)
1 tablespoon dried tarragon
2 teaspoons ground black pepper
1 teaspoon garlic powder

1.  Preheat oven to 300°F.
2.  Place chicken breasts on a rack in a large shallow pan. Bake, covered, 30 minutes, or until juices run clear and no longer pink inside. Remove from oven, cover, and let sit 10 minutes. Place in refrigerator to cool.

3. Meanwhile, bring 4 quarts water to boil in a large pot. Add pasta and cook according to package directions, until al dente, 5 to 7 minutes. Add frozen peas to cooking pasta 3 minutes before pasta is done; do not over-cook. Drain, set aside, and keep warm.
4. In a large bowl, combine sliced carrots, diced celery, and diced peppers.
5. In a small bowl, combine olive oil, lemon juice, mayonnaise, parsley, mustard, lemon rind, tarragon, pepper, and garlic powder. Stir well with a whisk.
6. Cut cooled chicken into 2-inch pieces and add to vegetables. Add pasta and peas and toss gently. Drizzle with dressing, toss, cover, and chill for 20 to 30 minutes.

SERVES 8

# Garden Salad

*Total preparation time: 10 minutes*

2 small heads red-leaf lettuce, outer leaves removed, washed, dried, and torn into bite-size pieces

2 small heads romaine, outer leaves removed, washed, dried, and torn into bite-size pieces

3 large cucumbers, peeled and thinly sliced

12 dozen radishes, washed, trimmed, and thinly sliced

4 large tomatoes, washed and quartered

½ cup fat-free salad dressing

In a large salad bowl, toss lettuces, cucumbers, radishes, and tomatoes. Dress immediately before serving.

SERVES 8

## Marinated Green Bean and Tomato Salad

*Total preparation time: 25 minutes*

**2 pounds fresh green beans, trimmed and washed**
**4 large tomatoes, washed and quartered**
**1 medium red onion, peeled and thinly sliced**
**½ cup fat-free vinaigrette or Italian salad dressing of choice**

1. Bring 2 inches water to boil in a large covered saucepan. Add green beans and cook until just tender but still bright green, 3 to 4 minutes. Drain and shock in cold water to halt cooking.
2. In a large mixing bowl, toss tomatoes, onions, and cooled green beans. Add dressing and stir gently to mix. Cover and marinate in refrigerator 15 minutes, or up to 1 hour. Serve chilled.

SERVES 8

## Herbed Yogurt Cheese

*Total preparation time: 24 hours to ferment yogurt, plus 10 minutes preparation\**

**3 cups plain nonfat yogurt**
**½ teaspoon garlic powder**
**½ teaspoon fresh lemon juice**
**1 scallion, trimmed and finely diced**
**½ teaspoon dried oregano**
**½ teaspoon ground black pepper**

1. Spoon yogurt into a coffee filter or cheesecloth-lined sieve and place over a small bowl. Cover with plastic wrap and refrigerate 24 hours. Discard liquid.
2. In a medium bowl, combine yogurt cheese, garlic powder, lemon juice,

scallion, oregano, and pepper; mix until blended. Serve as a spread on French bread or crackers.

SERVES 8

*Prepare this cheese spread one or two days ahead.

# Triple Berry Fruit Salad

*Total preparation time: 20 minutes*

1 quart strawberries, hulled, washed, and thinly sliced
1 pint blackberries or blueberries, washed, stems and debris removed
1 pint raspberries, washed
2 teaspoons lemon juice
2 tablespoons sugar

Combine all ingredients in medium bowl and stir gently. Cover and refrigerate 10 to 15 minutes. Serve chilled.

SERVES 8

NUTRITIONAL INFORMATION PER SERVING

|  | Calories | Protein | Carbohydrate | Fat | Fiber | Sodium | Cholesterol | Calcium |
|---|---|---|---|---|---|---|---|---|
| Chicken Bowtie Salad | 651 | 54 g | 62 g | 19 g (27%) | 8 g | 453 mg | 120 mg | 87 mg |
| Garden Salad | 59 | 3 g | 13 g | 0.5 g (6%) | 3 g | 177 mg | 0 mg | 62 mg |
| Marinated Green Bean and Tomato Salad | 61 | 2 g | 14 g | 0.5 g (5%) | 4 g | 186 mg | 0 mg | 49 mg |
| Herbed Yogurt Cheese | 65 | 5 g | 8 g | 1.5 g (20%) | 1 g | 67 mg | 6 mg | 172 mg |
| Triple Berry Fruit Salad | 57 | 1 g | 19 g | 0.5 g (3%) | 6 g | 1 mg | 0 mg | 23 mg |

## BACKYARD BARBECUE

**Grilled Salmon and Baked Potato with Salsa**
**Grilled Red Peppers with Roasted Corn Relish**
**Caesar Salad**
**Spinach–Stuffed Mushrooms**
**Assorted Melon Wedges**

# Grilled Salmon and Baked Potato with Salsa

*Total preparation time: 30 minutes*

8 medium baking potatoes (russet or Idaho), unpeeled and well scrubbed
Eight 7-ounce salmon steaks
⅔ tablespoon olive oil
2⅔ tablespoons Dijon mustard
½ cup nonfat sour cream
½ cup salsa

1. Prepare grill.
2. Prick each potato several times with a fork and wrap individually in aluminum foil. Place on grill 20 to 25 minutes, or until fork tender.
3. Meanwhile, brush salmon with olive oil and mustard. Grill 5 minutes on one side, turn, and continue grilling 5 to 7 minutes or until fish flakes easily to fork or is no longer translucent. Top each potato with 2 tablespoons each of sour cream and salsa, and serve with cooked fish.

SERVES 8

# Grilled Red Peppers with Roasted Corn Relish

*Total preparation time: 35 minutes*

3 cups fresh, canned, or frozen corn kernels (thawed and drained if frozen corn is used)

1 large red onion, peeled and finely diced

½ pound green peas, fresh or frozen (thawed and drained if frozen peas are used)

2 tablespoons granulated sugar

1 tablespoon olive oil

2 teaspoons dry mustard

2 teaspoons dried oregano

½ teaspoon ground black pepper

4 medium red bell peppers, washed, cored, seeded, and halved

4 ounces shredded reduced-fat Monterey Jack cheese

1. Prepare grill with rack 5 inches from coals.
2. In a large metal baking pan, combine corn, onion, peas, sugar, oil, mustard, oregano, and pepper; mix well. Place pan on grill rack, cover, and cook 15 minutes, stirring occasionally, until begins to brown.
3. Spoon relish evenly into pepper halves, and sprinkle with cheese. Arrange filled peppers in the baking pan, place on grill rack, cover, and cook 15 minutes, until peppers are tender and cheese is melted.

SERVES 8

# Caesar Salad

*Total preparation time: 20 minutes*

½ cup grated Parmesan cheese
½ cup fat-free mayonnaise
¼ cup lemon juice
1 teaspoon anchovy paste
1 teaspoon Worcestershire sauce
½ teaspoon freshly ground black pepper
¼ teaspoon dry mustard
4 cloves garlic, peeled and minced
½ loaf (8 ounces) sliced French bread, cut into ¾-inch cubes
4 heads romaine lettuce, outer leaves removed, washed, dried, and torn into
   bite-size pieces

1.   Preheat oven to 300°F.
2.   In a small bowl, combine ½ cup water with cheese, mayonnaise, lemon juice, anchovy paste, Worcestershire sauce, pepper, mustard, and garlic. Stir with a whisk and set aside.
3.   Place bread cubes on a cookie sheet and bake at 300°F 15 minutes or until toasted.
4.   In a large salad bowl, combine croutons and romaine. Dress immediately before serving.

SERVES 8

# Spinach-Stuffed Mushrooms

*Total preparation time: 40 minutes*

16 large button mushrooms, washed and dried
Nonstick cooking spray
¼ medium yellow onion, peeled and finely diced
2 cloves garlic, peeled and minced
One 10-ounce box frozen spinach, thawed and drained
⅓ cup dried bread crumbs
¼ cup egg substitute
1 tablespoon chopped fresh parsley
½ teaspoon dried oregano
¼ teaspoon salt
¼ teaspoon ground black pepper

1. Preheat oven to 350°F.
2. Remove stems from mushrooms. Discard the woody ends, and chop the stems. Set aside caps.
3. Lightly coat a large nonstick skillet with cooking spray and set over medium-high heat. Add chopped mushroom stems, onion, and garlic and sauté, stirring frequently, 5 minutes, or until tender. Add chopped spinach and cook until spinach is tender but still bright green, 5 minutes. Remove from heat and drain any excess moisture. Add bread crumbs, egg substitute, parsley, oregano, salt, and pepper, and mix well.
4. Lightly coat an 11-x-17-inch baking pan with nonstick cooking spray. Place mushroom caps in pan, and fill with equal portions of the stuffing mixture. Bake in 350°F oven 25 to 30 minutes, until lightly browned.

SERVES 8

NUTRITIONAL INFORMATION PER SERVING

| | Calories | Protein | Carbohydrate | Fat | Fiber | Sodium | Cholesterol | Calcium |
|---|---|---|---|---|---|---|---|---|
| **Grilled Salmon and Baked Potato with Salsa** | 521 | 51 g | 37 g | 18 g (31%) | 3 g | 309 mg | 97 mg | 125 mg |
| **Grilled Red Peppers with Corn Relish** | 150 | 8 g | 26 g | 3 g (15%) | 4 g | 340 mg | 2.5 mg | 226 mg |
| **Caesar Salad** | 88 | 5 g | 14 g | 2 g (15%) | 2 g | 361 mg | 4 mg | 110 mg |
| **Spinach-Stuffed Mushrooms** | 44 | 3 g | 7 g | 1 g (14%) | 1.5 g | 144 mg | 0 mg | 54 mg |

# WINTER HOLIDAY DINNER

**Chicken Breasts Provencale**
**Gingered Carrots**
**Boiled New Potatoes with Rosemary and Thyme**
**Chocolate Mocha Pudding**

# Chicken Breasts Provencale

*Total preparation time: 25 minutes*

1 large eggplant, cut into 2-inch cubes
4 medium tomatoes, washed, quartered, and thinly sliced
2 medium yellow onions, peeled, and thinly sliced
2 medium red bell peppers, washed, cored, seeded, and cut into thin strips
2 medium green peppers, washed, cored, seeded, and cut into thin strips
½ cup red or dry white wine (substitute chicken broth)
4 tablespoons chopped fresh basil *or* 1½ teaspoons dried
4 cloves garlic, peeled and minced
½ teaspoon salt

Eight 7-ounce boneless, skinless, chicken breasts (3½ pounds total)
2 tablespoons olive oil
1 teaspoon paprika

1.  In a large saucepan, combine eggplant, tomatoes, onions, red and green peppers, wine or chicken broth, basil, garlic, and salt. Bring to a boil, reduce heat to low, cover, and simmer 10 minutes; uncover and simmer 5 more minutes, or until vegetables are tender and nearly all of the liquid is evaporated.
2.  Meanwhile, rinse chicken and pat dry. Place each breast between 2 pieces of plastic wrap, and working from the center to the edges, pound chicken lightly with a meat mallet until ¼ inch thick. Remove plastic wrap.
3.  Heat oil and paprika in a large, nonstick skillet over medium-high flame. Add chicken and sauté 6 to 8 minutes, turning once, or until the chicken is tender and no longer pink inside.
4.  Spoon vegetables on top of chicken and serve.

SERVES 8

# Gingered Carrots

*Total preparation time: 25 minutes*

1 pound carrots, trimmed, peeled, cut into ½-inch slices
2 teaspoons olive oil
½ teaspoon ground ginger
1 teaspoon orange peel

1.  Place carrots in medium saucepan; add water to cover. Bring to a boil. Reduce heat and simmer, covered, for 15 minutes or until carrots are tender. Drain, cover, and keep warm.
2.  In a small bowl, blend olive oil, ginger, and orange peel. Drizzle over carrots, stirring gently, until carrots are well coated. Serve immediately.

SERVES 4

# Boiled New Potatoes with Rosemary and Thyme

*Total preparation time: 35 minutes*

2½ pounds small new or red bliss potatoes, well-scrubbed and cut into
   quarters
Nonstick cooking spray
4 cloves garlic, peeled and minced
½ teaspoon dried rosemary
½ teaspoon dried thyme
¾ cup low-sodium chicken broth

1.  Place potatoes in a large covered saucepan with enough water to cover.
    Bring to a boil, reduce heat to medium, and cook until potatoes are just
    slightly undercooked, 20 minutes. Drain and keep warm.
2.  Spray a large nonstick skillet with cooking spray. Add garlic, rosemary,
    and thyme, and cook over low heat, stirring constantly, 1 minute. Add
    potatoes and toss to coat. Add broth, increase heat to medium-high,
    cover, and cook 2 minutes. Remove cover and cook until liquid has evap-
    orated and potatoes are fork-tender, 7 to 8 minutes.

SERVES 8

# Chocolate Mocha Pudding

*Total preparation time: 10 minutes to prepare, 2 hours to set*

2 envelopes unflavored gelatin
2 cups skim milk
⅔ cup firmly packed dark brown sugar
1½ cups part-skim ricotta cheese
½ cup unsweetened cocoa powder
2⅔ tablespoons coffee liqueur

2 teaspoons vanilla extract
½ cup fat-free whipped topping
1 Slim•Fast Nutritional Snack Bar, grated

1.  In a small saucepan, sprinkle gelatin over milk; let stand 1 minute. Stir in brown sugar and cook over medium-low heat, stirring constantly, about 2 minutes, until gelatin is completely dissolved; do not boil.
2.  In a blender or food processor, combine ricotta, cocoa powder, coffee liqueur, and vanilla extract. Process on medium about 1 minute, until pureed, scraping down sides as necessary.
3.  Reduce speed to low and gradually add milk mixture. Process until combined.
4.  Evenly pour pudding into eight 6-ounce custard cups or parfait glasses. Cover with plastic wrap and refrigerate until set, at least 2 hours. Immediately before serving, garnish each portion with 2 tablespoons fat-free whipped topping and Slim•Fast Nutritional Snack Bar crumbles.

SERVES 8

NUTRITIONAL INFORMATION PER SERVING

|  | Calories | Protein | Carbohydrate | Fat | Fiber | Sodium | Cholesterol | Calcium |
|---|---|---|---|---|---|---|---|---|
| **Chicken Breasts Provencale** | 362 | 44 g | 10 g | 15 g (37%) | 3 g | 399 mg | 120 mg | 40 mg |
| **Gingered Carrots** | 70 | 1 g | 12 g | 2.5g (30%) | 3.5 g | 40 mg | 0 mg | 32 mg |
| **Boiled New Potatoes with Rosemary and Thyme** | 110 | 2.5 g | 25 g | 0.5 g (2%) | 2 g | 99 mg | 0 mg | 11 mg |
| **Chocolate Mocha Pudding** | 209 | 10 g | 30 g | 5.5g (23%) | 2 g | 111mg | 16 mg | 241 mg |

## THANKSGIVING

**Mushroom Bouillon**
**Roast Turkey with Sage Stuffing**
**Whole Cranberry Sauce**
**Sweet Potatoes with Apples**
**Green Beans with Rosemary**
**Sautéed Spinach and Onions**
**Pumpkin Pie Pudding**

# Mushroom Bouillon

*Total preparation time: 55 minutes*

3/4 **pound button mushrooms, washed, ends trimmed, and diced (reserve 3 unblemished mushrooms for garnish; cut into slices)**
**2 stalks celery, washed, trimmed, and diced**
**1 large carrot, peeled and diced**
**½ medium yellow onion, peeled and diced**
**¼ cup dry sherry**
**⅛ teaspoon freshly ground black pepper**
**5 cups low-sodium beef broth**

1. Place mushrooms, celery, carrot, onion, and 3 cups water in a large covered saucepan and bring to a boil. Reduce heat to low and simmer, partially covered, 45 minutes. Add sherry and pepper and simmer, uncovered, 2 minutes.
2. Strain through a fine-mesh sieve or strainer, pressing vegetables to extract as much juice as possible. Add beef broth and simmer until heated through. Serve in bouillon cups, garnished with reserved mushroom slices.

SERVES 8

# Roast Turkey with Sage Stuffing

*Total preparation time: 4½ hours*

1 large yellow onion, peeled and diced
2 stalks celery, washed, trimmed, and diced
2 cups chicken broth
1 teaspoon dried sage
1 teaspoon dried marjoram
1 teaspoon dried thyme
½ teaspoon ground black pepper
8 slices stale white or whole-wheat bread, cut into cubes
One 12-pound whole turkey
1 tablespoon diet margarine

1.  Preheat oven to 325°F.
2.  Place onion, celery, and chicken broth in a large covered saucepan and simmer until onions and celery are tender, 20 minutes. Add sage, marjoram, thyme, and pepper.
3.  Place bread cubes in a large bowl, pour broth mixture over, and gently mix until thoroughly combined.
4.  Rinse turkey under cool water, drain thoroughly, and pat dry. Fill the neck pocket and body cavity loosely with stuffing. Secure neck flap and body cavity with skewers; tie wings and legs close to body with string. Rub margarine over breast and legs.
5.  Place turkey, breast side up, in a shallow roasting pan. Cover lightly with aluminum foil or cheesecloth that has been dampened, and roast approximately 18 minutes per pound, or 3½ hours. Remove foil or cheesecloth during the last hour to allow bird to brown. The turkey is done when a meat thermometer inserted to the center of the inside thigh muscle, not touching bone, registers 185°F. Remove from roasting pan to a heated platter, cover with foil, and let rest in a warm place 30 minutes before serving.

SERVES 8, WITH LEFTOVERS

# Whole Cranberry Sauce

*Total preparation time: 4 hours, 15 minutes (includes 4 hours to gel in refrigerator)*

**One 7-gram packet unflavored gelatin**
**12 ounces orange juice**
**12 ounces cranberries, washed**
**1 teaspoon grated orange rind, orange part only (no white pith)**
**Three 1-gram packets sugar substitute**

1. In a small saucepan, sprinkle gelatin over 4 ounces of the orange juice; let stand 1 minute. Stir over low heat until dissolved.
2. Place cranberries and 1 cup of the orange juice in a medium covered saucepan and bring to boil. Cover and boil 3 minutes, or until the berry skins burst. Remove from heat, gradually add gelatin mixture, and stir in grated orange rind and sugar substitute. Pour into a mold or clear bowl and chill 4 hours or more. Serve chilled.

SERVES 8

# Sweet Potatoes with Apples

*Total preparation time: 1 hour*

**3 large Cortland or McIntosh apples, skin-on, washed, cored, and thinly
  sliced**
**1 tablespoon lemon juice**
**Nonstick cooking spray**
**1½ pounds sweet potatoes, peeled, and cut into ½-inch slices**
**¼ cup apple cider**

1. Preheat oven to 350°F.
2. Place apples in a mixing bowl and coat with lemon juice.
3. Lightly coat a large casserole dish with cooking spray. Layer potatoes and
   apples in casserole and pour cider over all. Cover with aluminum foil and
   bake in 350°F oven 40 minutes. Uncover and continue to bake 15 minutes,
   or until potatoes are fork tender.

SERVES 8

# Green Beans with Rosemary

*Total preparation time: 15 minutes*

**2 pounds fresh green beans, trimmed, washed, and cut into 2-inch pieces**
**2 tablespoons chopped fresh rosemary**
**1 teaspoon olive oil**

Bring 1 inch water to boil in a medium saucepan. Add beans and cook, uncovered, 5 minutes. Cover, reduce heat to low, add rosemary, and continue cooking 2 to 3 minutes, until beans are crisp-tender but still bright green. Drain,
place in a serving bowl, add olive oil, and gently toss to coat.

SERVES 8

# Sautéed Spinach and Onions

*Total preparation time: 15 minutes*

Nonstick cooking spray
1 tablespoon olive oil
1 medium yellow onion, peeled and diced
2 cloves garlic, peeled and minced
Two 10-ounce packages fresh spinach, stems removed, washed well, and
    coarsely chopped
1/8 teaspoon ground black pepper

1.  Spray a large nonstick skillet or saucepan with cooking spray, brush with oil, and set over medium-high heat. Add onions and garlic and sauté, stirring frequently, until onions wilt, 1 to 2 minutes.
2.  Add spinach, cover, reduce heat to low, and cook, stirring frequently, until spinach is wilted but still bright green, 3 to 4 minutes. Remove pan from heat, stir in pepper, and serve.

SERVES 8

# Pumpkin Pie Pudding

*Total preparation time: 40 minutes*

Two 11-ounce cans French Vanilla Ultra Slim•Fast Ready-to-Drink Shake
2 packets unflavored gelatin
3/4 cup canned pumpkin
1 teaspoon vanilla extract
1 tablespoon maple syrup
1/4 teaspoon ground cinnamon
1 cup light whipped topping
1/4 teaspoon ground nutmeg

1.   Place ½ can Ultra Slim•Fast shake in a small saucepan, sprinkle gelatin on top, and let sit 1 minute to soften gelatin.
2.   Meanwhile, combine the remaining 1½ cans Slim•Fast with the pumpkin, vanilla, maple syrup, and cinnamon in blender or food processor. Blend for 30 seconds.
3.   Heat the saucepan of gelatin- Slim•Fast mixture over medium flame, stirring constantly, until gelatin dissolves, 1 minute. Add the warmed gelatin mixture to the pumpkin mixture in the blender and process 30 seconds.
4.   Pour into individual custard cups or parfait glasses and chill 30 minutes. Garnish each with 2 tablespoons whipped topping and a dash of nutmeg. Serve very cold.

SERVES 8

NUTRITIONAL INFORMATION PER SERVING

|  | Calories | Protein | Carbohydrate | Fat | Fiber | Sodium | Cholesterol | Calcium |
|---|---|---|---|---|---|---|---|---|
| Mushroom Bouillon | 48 | 4 g | 4.5 g | 1 g (20%) | 1 g | 59 mg | 0 mg | 17 mg |
| Roast Turkey with Sage Stuffing | 319 | 54 g | 13 g | 4 g (12%) | 1 g | 491 mg | 142 mg | 54 mg |
| Whole Cranberry Sauce | 43 | 1 g | 10 g | 0.5 g (3%) | 2 g | 3 mg | 0 mg | 9 mg |
| Sweet Potatoes with Apples | 104 | 1 g | 26 g | 0.5 g (3%) | 4 g | 5 mg | 0 mg | 21 mg |
| Green Beans with Rosemary | 41 | 2 g | 8 g | 1 g (17%) | 3 g | 3 mg | 0 mg | 51 mg |
| Sautéed Spinach and onions | 24 | 2 g | 5 g | 2 g (38%) | 5 g | 61 mg | 0 mg | 43 mg |
| Pumpkin Pie Pudding | 116 | 4 g | 20 g | 2 g (14%) | 3 g | 171 mg | 1 mg | 113 mg |

# Cocktail Party Menu
# New Year's Eve Cocktail Party

Smoked Salmon Canapés
Zucchini Pizzas
Spinach Dip with Crudités
Cocktail Meatballs with Sweet-and-Sour Sauce
Baba Ghanouj with Pita Triangles
Strawberries with Chocolate Dipping Sauce

## Smoked Salmon Canapés

*Total preparation time: 10 minutes*

4 ounces smoked salmon
8 ounces light cream cheese
16 slices party-size pumpernickel bread
¼ cup fresh dill

1.  Cut smoked salmon into 1-inch pieces.
2.  Spread a thin layer of cream cheese on cocktail bread. Place a piece of salmon on top of each bread slice. Slice in half, diagonally, to form 2 triangles, and garnish with dill. Place on serving tray, cover with plastic wrap, and refrigerate until ready to serve.

SERVES 8

# Zucchini Pizzas

*Total preparation time: 10 minutes*

2 medium zucchini, washed and cut into ¼-inch slices
1 cup pizza sauce
4 ounces fat-free mozzarella cheese, shredded
½ medium green bell pepper, washed, cored, seeded, and finely diced
12 medium pitted black olives, chopped

1.  Preheat broiler.
2.  Place zucchini on baking sheet. Top each piece with sauce, cheese, diced
    green pepper, and black olives. Broil until cheese is melted and bubbly, 3
    to 4 minutes. Serve immediately.

SERVES 8

# Spinach Dip with Crudités

*Very attractive when served in a hollowed-out red cabbage.*
*Total preparation time: 1 hour, 10 minutes (includes 1 hour chilling time in refrigerator)*

One 10-ounce bag fresh spinach, stems trimmed, well washed
1 cup low-fat (1%) cottage cheese
1 tablespoon lemon juice
½ cup fat-free mayonnaise
1 cup plain nonfat yogurt
2 tablespoons chopped fresh parsley
2 tablespoons chopped fresh chives
1 tablespoon Mrs. Dash seasoning
1 large head red cabbage
6 large romaine lettuce leaves, washed and dried
Crudités (recipe below)

1.  Place spinach in a medium covered saucepan with 2 inches water and set over high heat. Bring to a boil, reduce heat to medium, and simmer, covered, 3 minutes, until wilted. Remove from heat and drain thoroughly, squeezing out excess moisture. Coarsely chop and set aside.
2.  In a blender or food processor, process cottage cheese with lemon juice until well-mixed. Add mayonnaise, yogurt, parsley, chives, Mrs. Dash, and cooked spinach, and process until just mixed.
3.  Cover and refrigerate 1 hour or up to 24 hours to blend flavors.
4.  Meanwhile, flatten bottom of the cabbage head by slicing off a piece so it will sit straight. With a sharp knife, carefully carve out inside of cabbage; use a smaller paring knife to scoop out insides.
5.  Lay a bed of lettuce leaves on a larger platter and place cabbage in the center. Fill with the chilled dip and surround with crudités.

SERVES 8

## Crudités (Fresh Vegetables)

*Total preparation time: 15 minutes*

1 pound broccoli, tough ends removed, washed and cut into florets
1 pound cauliflower, tough ends removed, washed and cut into florets
2 large red bell peppers, washed, cored, seeded, and cut into thin strips
4 celery stalks, washed, trimmed, strings removed, and cut into thin strips
½ pound carrots, trimmed, peeled, and cut into thin strips

Arrange raw vegetables around dip on platter. Serve immediately.

SERVES 8

# Cocktail Meatballs with Sweet-and-Sour Sauce

*Total preparation time: 35 minutes*

½ pound extra-lean ground beef
½ pound ground turkey breast, without skin
¼ cup egg substitute
¼ cup bread crumbs
½ teaspoon Worcestershire sauce
¼ teaspoon black pepper
½ small yellow onion, peeled, diced fine
1 cup ketchup
1 tablespoon brown sugar
1 tablespoon lemon juice

1.  Preheat oven to 350°F.
2.  Combine beef, turkey, egg, bread crumbs, Worcestershire sauce, and pepper in a large bowl and mix well. Shape into 16 to 20 meatballs, place on a baking tray, and cook 20 minutes, or until no longer pink inside (cut one meatball in half to test). Remove from tray and place on paper towel–lined plate to drain off excess fat.
3.  Meanwhile, place diced onion, ketchup, sugar, and lemon juice in a large covered saucepan over medium-low heat. Simmer 3 to 4 minutes to blend flavors, add drained meatballs, and continue to cook 5 minutes. Serve warm with toothpicks.

SERVES 8

# Baba Ghanouj with Pita Triangles

*Total preparation time: 1 hour 40 minutes*

2 medium eggplants, halved

⅓ cup lemon juice

¼ cup tahini (sesame seed paste)

4 cloves garlic, peeled and minced

¼ teaspoon salt

¼ teaspoon freshly ground black pepper

⅓ cup chopped fresh parsley

6 ounces pita bread, cut into triangles

1 large red onion, peeled, quartered, and layers separated

1. Preheat broiler.
2. Place eggplants, cut side down, on a cookie sheet 8 inches from heat. Gently pierce eggplant with a fork and broil until skin starts to brown and eggplant becomes soft inside, 30 minutes.
3. Cool eggplants, gently scoop out meat, and separate from skin. Place meat in a blender or food processor with ¼ of the charred skin, and add lemon juice, tahini, garlic, salt, and pepper; blend or pulse until smooth. Scoop into a serving bowl, garnish with parsley, cover, and chill at least 1 hour, or up to overnight.
4. To serve, place bowl on a serving platter and surround with pita triangles and red onion pieces.

SERVES 8

# Strawberries with Chocolate Dipping Sauce

*Total preparation time: 10 minutes*

½ cup fat-free milk
½ cup chocolate yogurt
1 scoop Ultra Slim•Fast Chocolate Royale powder
24 large (1 quart) fresh strawberries, hulled and washed

In a blender, combine milk, yogurt, and Ultra Slim•Fast, and process until smooth. Place in small bowl in the center of a serving platter, and surround with strawberries. Cover and chill until ready to serve.

SERVES 8

NUTRITIONAL INFORMATION PER SERVING

|  | Calories | Protein | Carbohydrate | Fat | Fiber | Sodium | Cholesterol | Calcium |
|---|---|---|---|---|---|---|---|---|
| Smoked Salmon Canapés | 130 | 10 g | 16 g | 4 g (27%) | 2 g | 489 mg | 13 mg | 48 mg |
| Zucchini Pizzas | 58 | 5 g | 5 g | 2 g (25%) | 1 g | 250 mg | 3 mg | 220 mg |
| Spinach Dip with Crudités | 87 | 8 g | 15 g | 1 g (10%) | 4 g | 445 mg | 4 mg | 130 mg |
| Cocktail Meatballs with Sweet-and-Sour Sauce | 148 | 15 g | 14 g | 4 g (23%) | 1 g | 445 mg | 31 mg | 28 mg |
| Baba Ghanouj with Pita Triangles | 152 | 5 g | 25 g | 5 g (27%) | 5 g | 193 mg | 0 mg | 46 mg |
| Strawberries with Chocolate Dipping Sauce | 65 | 2 g | 12 g | 1 g ( 13%) | 3 g | 35 mg | 2 mg | 77 mg |

# 10

# MAINTAINING
# YOUR MAKEOVER

If you've given yourself the Body•Mind•Life Makeover, you've given your-self a great gift. You've improved your health and weight. You've improved the physical fitness of your body and the spiritual fitness of your mind. You've taken charge of your life to make each day more fulfilling than the day before. As you continue in the coming weeks and months, you're in the perfect position to transform your life for good.

This book may be coming to an end, but your makeover is just beginning. As you'll see, it will continue to evolve as you lose weight and gain the energy to do things you never thought possible. You'll probably want to try new fit-ness activities, to travel to new places, to update your look and your wardrobe. You'll crave excitement from your life, and start looking for new adventures. If you allow this sense of freshness and excitement to refresh you every day, you should have no trouble staying on the makeover plan.

If you've been concerned about improving your health, the makeover will continue to help. Maintaining a healthy weight can help prevent many of the diseases associated with the aging process. You'll have a lower risk of developing heart disease, diabetes, and certain cancers. The combination of exercising and eating a nutritious, calcium-rich, well-balanced diet that includes Slim•Fast can help stave off osteoporosis and keep your immune sys-tem finely tuned. Your body will thank you, and you'll continue to feel and look better than you ever have in your life.

At some point along the way, you should reach a weight you're happy with and feel satisfied with your fitness level. You'll probably think to yourself, "I feel good staying just where I am." It's at this point that you may be tempted to revert back to your old ways; after all, we live in a goal-oriented society, and we're used to putting forth effort just long enough to receive our rewards.

If you find yourself slipping back into your old habits, think about how you've been feeling lately. Do you have less energy? Are you feeling bloated and out of sorts? Are your pants feeling tighter? Remember the point of the Body•Mind•Life Makeover: to infuse you with good health, energy, and vitality. If you abandon the makeover, your body will let you know. You'll also find your weight creeping back up the scale. The truth is, unless you follow the healthy principles you've learned, it won't take long for your body to revert to its old shape.

Remember, in order to maintain a weight loss, you need to eat far fewer calories than you ate at your old weight. The best way to do this is to follow the nutrition plan and replace one meal a day with a Slim•Fast product—especially if you find yourself gaining weight. Don't allow yourself to get into a meal rut (if it's Tuesday, it must be salmon). Use the dozens of recipes throughout this book to vary your cooking and keep your taste buds tantalized. And make an effort to try new fruits and vegetables—like grape tomatoes, yellow plums, or broccolini—that catch your eye in the supermarket. The best way to stick with any plan, after all, is to keep it interesting.

You should also take measures to avoid boredom with your fitness program. The minute you feel you're no longer being challenged, increase the intensity or duration of your workouts, or switch to a new activity altogether. If you've pedaled too many miles on the stationary bike or climbed too many stairs on the stair machine, try taking a step or kick-boxing class. If you've worn down the path that takes you around your neighborhood, find a new walking route that challenges you with hills. The more you can make over your makeover as you go, the better off you'll be.

You may even find that you need to revamp your relaxation plan from time to time. You should feel invigorated, not bored, after practicing your technique. Feel free to try a new technique if you find your old one is putting you to sleep rather than relaxing you.

As you can see, the Body•Mind•Life Makeover has fail-safes that should keep you from getting bored with the plan. There are so many eating, exercise, and relaxation options here that you can re-create your plan every couple of weeks. The key is to try out new options once you find that you're getting stuck in a rut.

To gauge how you're doing on your makeover, you need to continue to fill in your makeover diary *every day*. Read through your diary every week to get a quick assessment of how you feel on the plan. At the beginning of each week, think about what is or isn't working for you, and then implement new options to keep your plan fresh.

At certain times you'll probably be more faithful to the makeover plan than at others. Don't beat yourself up or sit in judgment of yourself if you cheat a little! Just remember how great you feel when you're sticking with your plan, and use that as a motivation to get back on track. Feeling guilty is self-defeating, and can actually cause you to lose faith. Whatever you do, *never* let yourself think "Oh, what the heck—I've already blown it." It ain't over till it's over—till you have the life you want.

As the saying goes, *Today is the first day of the rest of your life*. Make today the day you begin anew—whether you're beginning your makeover for the first time or renewing your commitment to the plan. Here's to you and your new life!

*Lauren Hutton*

# YOUR PERSONAL MAKEOVER DIARY

## WEEK 1

● **Sunday**

Daily Weigh-in: _____

Breakfast: _____

Snack: _____

Lunch: _____

Snack: _____

Snack: _____

Dinner: _____

Estimated Calorie Intake: _____

Activity: _____

Estimated Calorie Burn: _____

Relaxation Technique: _____

General Comments About How You Feel: _____

● **Monday**

Daily Weigh-in: _____

Breakfast: _____

Snack: _____

Lunch: _____

Snack: _____

Snack: _____

Dinner: _____

Estimated Calorie Intake: _____

Activity: _____

Estimated Calorie Burn: _____

Relaxation Technique: _____

General Comments About How You Feel: _____

# YOUR PERSONAL MAKEOVER DIARY

## WEEK 1

### ● Tuesday

Daily Weigh-in: _____

Breakfast: _____

Snack: _____

Lunch: _____

Snack: _____

Snack: _____

Dinner: _____

Estimated Calorie Intake: _____

Activity: _____

Estimated Calorie Burn: _____

Relaxation Technique: _____

General Comments About How You Feel: _____

### ● Wednesday

Daily Weigh-in: _____

Breakfast: _____

Snack: _____

Lunch: _____

Snack: _____

Snack: _____

Dinner: _____

Estimated Calorie Intake: _____

Activity: _____

Estimated Calorie Burn: _____

Relaxation Technique: _____

General Comments About How You Feel: _____

# YOUR PERSONAL MAKEOVER DIARY

## WEEK 1

● **Thursday**

Daily Weigh-in: _____

Breakfast: _____

Snack: _____

Lunch: _____

Snack: _____

Snack: _____

Dinner: _____

Estimated Calorie Intake: _____

Activity: _____

Estimated Calorie Burn: _____

Relaxation Technique: _____

General Comments About How You Feel: _____

● **Friday**

Daily Weigh-in: _____

Breakfast: _____

Snack: _____

Lunch: _____

Snack: _____

Snack: _____

Dinner: _____

Estimated Calorie Intake: _____

Activity: _____

Estimated Calorie Burn: _____

Relaxation Technique: _____

General Comments About How You Feel: _____

## WEEK 1

● **Saturday**

Daily Weigh-in: _____

Breakfast: _____

Snack: _____

Lunch: _____

Snack: _____

Snack: _____

Dinner: _____

Estimated Calorie Intake: _____

Activity: _____

Estimated Calorie Burn: _____

Relaxation Technique: _____

General Comments About How You Feel: _____

# YOUR PERSONAL MAKEOVER DIARY

● **Sunday**

Daily Weigh-in: _____

Breakfast: _____

Snack: _____

Lunch: _____

Snack: _____

Snack: _____

Dinner: _____

Estimated Calorie Intake: _____

Activity: _____

Estimated Calorie Burn: _____

Relaxation Technique: _____

General Comments About How You Feel: _____

● **Monday**

Daily Weigh-in: _____

Breakfast: _____

Snack: _____

Lunch: _____

Snack: _____

Snack: _____

Dinner: _____

Estimated Calorie Intake: _____

Activity: _____

Estimated Calorie Burn: _____

Relaxation Technique: _____

General Comments About How You Feel: _____

# YOUR PERSONAL MAKEOVER DIARY

## WEEK 2

### ● Tuesday

Daily Weigh-in: _____

Breakfast: _____

Snack: _____

Lunch: _____

Snack: _____

Snack: _____

Dinner: _____

Estimated Calorie Intake: _____

Activity: _____

Estimated Calorie Burn: _____

Relaxation Technique: _____

General Comments About How You Feel: _____

### ● Wednesday

Daily Weigh-in: _____

Breakfast: _____

Snack: _____

Lunch: _____

Snack: _____

Snack: _____

Dinner: _____

Estimated Calorie Intake: _____

Activity: _____

Estimated Calorie Burn: _____

Relaxation Technique: _____

General Comments About How You Feel: _____

# YOUR PERSONAL MAKEOVER DIARY

- **Thursday**

Daily Weigh-in: _____

Breakfast: _____

Snack: _____

Lunch: _____

Snack: _____

Snack: _____

Dinner: _____

Estimated Calorie Intake: _____

Activity: _____

Estimated Calorie Burn: _____

Relaxation Technique: _____

General Comments About How You Feel: _____

- **Friday**

Daily Weigh-in: _____

Breakfast: _____

Snack: _____

Lunch: _____

Snack: _____

Snack: _____

Dinner: _____

Estimated Calorie Intake: _____

Activity: _____

Estimated Calorie Burn: _____

Relaxation Technique: _____

General Comments About How You Feel: _____

# YOUR PERSONAL MAKEOVER DIARY

## WEEK 2

● **Saturday**

Daily Weigh-in: _____

Breakfast: _____

Snack: _____

Lunch: _____

Snack: _____

Snack: _____

Dinner: _____

Estimated Calorie Intake: _____

Activity: _____

Estimated Calorie Burn: _____

Relaxation Technique: _____

General Comments About How You Feel: _____

# YOUR PERSONAL MAKEOVER DIARY

## WEEK 3

● **Sunday**

Daily Weigh-in: _____

Breakfast: _____

Snack: _____

Lunch: _____

Snack: _____

Snack: _____

Dinner: _____

Estimated Calorie Intake: _____

Activity: _____

Estimated Calorie Burn: _____

Relaxation Technique: _____

General Comments About How You Feel: _____

● **Monday**

Daily Weigh-in: _____

Breakfast: _____

Snack: _____

Lunch: _____

Snack: _____

Snack: _____

Dinner: _____

Estimated Calorie Intake: _____

Activity: _____

Estimated Calorie Burn: _____

Relaxation Technique: _____

General Comments About How You Feel: _____

# YOUR PERSONAL MAKEOVER DIARY

## WEEK 3

### ● Tuesday

Daily Weigh-in: _____

Breakfast: _____

Snack: _____

Lunch: _____

Snack: _____

Snack: _____

Dinner: _____

Estimated Calorie Intake: _____

Activity: _____

Estimated Calorie Burn: _____

Relaxation Technique: _____

General Comments About How You Feel: _____

### ● Wednesday

Daily Weigh-in: _____

Breakfast: _____

Snack: _____

Lunch: _____

Snack: _____

Snack: _____

Dinner: _____

Estimated Calorie Intake: _____

Activity: _____

Estimated Calorie Burn: _____

Relaxation Technique: _____

General Comments About How You Feel: _____

# YOUR PERSONAL MAKEOVER DIARY

● **Thursday**

Daily Weigh-in: _____

Breakfast: _____

Snack: _____

Lunch: _____

Snack: _____

Snack: _____

Dinner: _____

Estimated Calorie Intake: _____

Activity: _____

Estimated Calorie Burn: _____

Relaxation Technique: _____

General Comments About How You Feel: _____

● **Friday**

Daily Weigh-in: _____

Breakfast: _____

Snack: _____

Lunch: _____

Snack: _____

Snack: _____

Dinner: _____

Estimated Calorie Intake: _____

Activity: _____

Estimated Calorie Burn: _____

Relaxation Technique: _____

General Comments About How You Feel: _____

## WEEK 3

● **Saturday**

Daily Weigh-in: _____

Breakfast: _____

Snack: _____

Lunch: _____

Snack: _____

Snack: _____

Dinner: _____

Estimated Calorie Intake: _____

Activity: _____

Estimated Calorie Burn: _____

Relaxation Technique: _____

General Comments About How You Feel: _____

# YOUR PERSONAL MAKEOVER DIARY

## WEEK 4

● **Sunday**

Daily Weigh-in: _____

Breakfast: _____

Snack: _____

Lunch: _____

Snack: _____

Snack: _____

Dinner: _____

Estimated Calorie Intake: _____

Activity: _____

Estimated Calorie Burn: _____

Relaxation Technique: _____

General Comments About How You Feel: _____

● **Monday**

Daily Weigh-in: _____

Breakfast: _____

Snack: _____

Lunch: _____

Snack: _____

Snack: _____

Dinner: _____

Estimated Calorie Intake: _____

Activity: _____

Estimated Calorie Burn: _____

Relaxation Technique: _____

General Comments About How You Feel: _____

# YOUR PERSONAL MAKEOVER DIARY

## WEEK 4

### ● Tuesday

Daily Weigh-in: _____

Breakfast: _____

Snack: _____

Lunch: _____

Snack: _____

Snack: _____

Dinner: _____

Estimated Calorie Intake: _____

Activity: _____

Estimated Calorie Burn: _____

Relaxation Technique: _____

General Comments About How You Feel: _____

### ● Wednesday

Daily Weigh-in: _____

Breakfast: _____

Snack: _____

Lunch: _____

Snack: _____

Snack: _____

Dinner: _____

Estimated Calorie Intake: _____

Activity: _____

Estimated Calorie Burn: _____

Relaxation Technique: _____

General Comments About How You Feel: _____

# YOUR PERSONAL MAKEOVER DIARY

## WEEK 4

● **Thursday**

Daily Weigh-in: _____

Breakfast: _____

Snack: _____

Lunch: _____

Snack: _____

Snack: _____

Dinner: _____

Estimated Calorie Intake: _____

Activity: _____

Estimated Calorie Burn: _____

Relaxation Technique: _____

General Comments About How You Feel: _____

● **Friday**

Daily Weigh-in: _____

Breakfast: _____

Snack: _____

Lunch: _____

Snack: _____

Snack: _____

Dinner: _____

Estimated Calorie Intake: _____

Activity: _____

Estimated Calorie Burn: _____

Relaxation Technique: _____

General Comments About How You Feel: _____

# YOUR PERSONAL MAKEOVER DIARY

## WEEK 4

● **Saturday**

Daily Weigh-in: _____

Breakfast: _____

Snack: _____

Lunch: _____

Snack: _____

Snack: _____

Dinner: _____

Estimated Calorie Intake: _____

Activity: _____

Estimated Calorie Burn: _____

Relaxation Technique: _____

General Comments About How You Feel: _____

# YOUR PERSONAL MAKEOVER DIARY

## WEEK 5

● **Sunday**

Daily Weigh-in: _____

Breakfast: _____

Snack: _____

Lunch: _____

Snack: _____

Snack: _____

Dinner: _____

Estimated Calorie Intake: _____

Activity: _____

Estimated Calorie Burn: _____

Relaxation Technique: _____

General Comments About How You Feel: _____

● **Monday**

Daily Weigh-in: _____

Breakfast: _____

Snack: _____

Lunch: _____

Snack: _____

Snack: _____

Dinner: _____

Estimated Calorie Intake: _____

Activity: _____

Estimated Calorie Burn: _____

Relaxation Technique: _____

General Comments About How You Feel: _____

# YOUR PERSONAL MAKEOVER DIARY

## WEEK 5

● **Tuesday**

Daily Weigh-in: _____

Breakfast: _____

Snack: _____

Lunch: _____

Snack: _____

Snack: _____

Dinner: _____

Estimated Calorie Intake: _____

Activity: _____

Estimated Calorie Burn: _____

Relaxation Technique: _____

General Comments About How You Feel: _____

● **Wednesday**

Daily Weigh-in: _____

Breakfast: _____

Snack: _____

Lunch: _____

Snack: _____

Snack: _____

Dinner: _____

Estimated Calorie Intake: _____

Activity: _____

Estimated Calorie Burn: _____

Relaxation Technique: _____

General Comments About How You Feel: _____

## WEEK 5

● **Thursday**

Daily Weigh-in: _____

Breakfast: _____

Snack: _____

Lunch: _____

Snack: _____

Snack: _____

Dinner: _____

Estimated Calorie Intake: _____

Activity: _____

Estimated Calorie Burn: _____

Relaxation Technique: _____

General Comments About How You Feel: _____

● **Friday**

Daily Weigh-in: _____

Breakfast: _____

Snack: _____

Lunch: _____

Snack: _____

Snack: _____

Dinner: _____

Estimated Calorie Intake: _____

Activity: _____

Estimated Calorie Burn: _____

Relaxation Technique: _____

General Comments About How You Feel: _____

# YOUR PERSONAL MAKEOVER DIARY

## WEEK 5

### • Saturday

Daily Weigh-in: _____

Breakfast: _____

Snack: _____

Lunch: _____

Snack: _____

Snack: _____

Dinner: _____

Estimated Calorie Intake: _____

Activity: _____

Estimated Calorie Burn: _____

Relaxation Technique: _____

General Comments About How You Feel: _____

# YOUR PERSONAL MAKEOVER DIARY

## WEEK 6

### ● Sunday

Daily Weigh-in: _____

Breakfast: _____

Snack: _____

Lunch: _____

Snack: _____

Snack: _____

Dinner: _____

Estimated Calorie Intake: _____

Activity: _____

Estimated Calorie Burn: _____

Relaxation Technique: _____

General Comments About How You Feel: _____

### ● Monday

Daily Weigh-in: _____

Breakfast: _____

Snack: _____

Lunch: _____

Snack: _____

Snack: _____

Dinner: _____

Estimated Calorie Intake: _____

Activity: _____

Estimated Calorie Burn: _____

Relaxation Technique: _____

General Comments About How You Feel: _____

# YOUR PERSONAL MAKEOVER DIARY

## WEEK 6

● **Tuesday**

Daily Weigh-in: _____

Breakfast: _____

Snack: _____

Lunch: _____

Snack: _____

Snack: _____

Dinner: _____

Estimated Calorie Intake: _____

Activity: _____

Estimated Calorie Burn: _____

Relaxation Technique: _____

General Comments About How You Feel: _____

● **Wednesday**

Daily Weigh-in: _____

Breakfast: _____

Snack: _____

Lunch: _____

Snack: _____

Snack: _____

Dinner: _____

Estimated Calorie Intake: _____

Activity: _____

Estimated Calorie Burn: _____

Relaxation Technique: _____

General Comments About How You Feel: _____

# YOUR PERSONAL MAKEOVER DIARY

## WEEK 6

### ● Thursday

Daily Weigh-in: _____

Breakfast: _____

Snack: _____

Lunch: _____

Snack: _____

Snack: _____

Dinner: _____

Estimated Calorie Intake: _____

Activity: _____

Estimated Calorie Burn: _____

Relaxation Technique: _____

General Comments About How You Feel: _____

### ● Friday

Daily Weigh-in: _____

Breakfast: _____

Snack: _____

Lunch: _____

Snack: _____

Snack: _____

Dinner: _____

Estimated Calorie Intake: _____

Activity: _____

Estimated Calorie Burn: _____

Relaxation Technique: _____

General Comments About How You Feel: _____

## WEEK 6

● **Saturday**

Daily Weigh-in: _____

Breakfast: _____

Snack: _____

Lunch: _____

Snack: _____

Snack: _____

Dinner: _____

Estimated Calorie Intake: _____

Activity: _____

Estimated Calorie Burn: _____

Relaxation Technique: _____

General Comments About How You Feel: _____

# Index